Caregiving

Caregiving

A Step-by-Step Resource for Caring for the Person with Cancer at Home

REVISED EDITION

Editors
Peter S. Houts, PhD
Julia A. Bucher, RN, PhD

Contributors
Arthur M. Nezu, PhD · Christine M. Nezu, PhD · Allan Lipton, MD · Harold A. Harvey, MD
Mary A. Simmonds, MD · Joan F. Hermann, LSW · Matthew J. Loscalzo, MSW
James R. Zabora, MSW, ScD · Dale B. Schelzel, RN, OCN · Sandra J. Spoljaric, RN, OCN
Kathy B. Kambic, RN, OCN · Elise M. Givant, RN, OCN · Georgia Brown, RN, OCN
Glenda M. Trumpower, MSW · Carol D. Nolt, MSW · Carole A. Bean

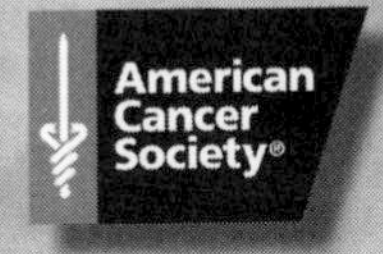

Printed in the United States of America

06 05 04 03 02 1 2 3 4 5

Library of Congress Cataloging in Publication Data

American Cancer Society's caregiving : a step-by-step resource for caring for people with cancer at home / editors, Peter S. Houts, Julia A. Bucher.-- Rev. ed.
p. ; cm.
Rev. ed. of: Caregiving. ©2000.
Includes index.
ISBN 0-944235-45-X (pbk. : alk. paper)
1. Cancer--Palliative treatment. 2. Cancer--Patients--Home care. 3. Caregivers.
[DNLM: 1. Home Nursing--methods--Popular Works. 2. Neoplasms--nursing--Popular Works. WY 200 A5115 2003] I. Title: Caregiving. II. Houts, Peter S. III. Bucher, Julia A. IV. American Cancer Society.

RC271.P33C37 2003
649'.8--dc21

2003001115

Managing Editor: Gianna Marsella, MA
Editor: Anneke Smith
Copy Editor: Tom Gryczan, MS
Book Publishing Manager: Candace Magee
Director, Publishing: Diane Scott-Lichter, MA
Editorial Review Board: Terri Ades, RN, Ted Gansler, MD; Peggy Pierce, MSN, MPH
Line illustrations: Charles H. Boyter, CMI; Mason Wiest, MSMI

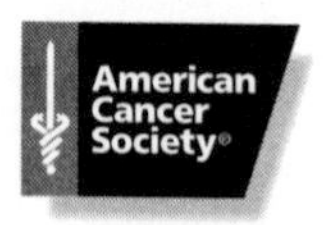

American Cancer Society
800-ACS-2345
www.cancer.org

Acknowledgments

Many people have contributed to the development of this book. They include physicians, nurses, psychologists, and social workers, as well as people with cancer and their family and friends. Several individuals have been especially generous in contributing their time and expertise and, as a result, have had a substantial influence on the development and growth of this project. We are deeply indebted to Regena Tripp, RN, OCN; David Houts; Charles Schreiber; Bruce Nicholson, MD; George Simms, MD; and the Cancer Control Program of the Pennsylvania Department of Health.

The chapters were reviewed and edited by cancer care professionals as well as by survivors. Their comments and editing have been invaluable. These include James B. Ray, PharmD; Kathleen Rine, RN, MSN; Deborah Clark, RN, BSN; Linda Mogul, MSW; Phyllis Hall, MSW; Mary Ann Cegielsky, RN, MSN, OCN; Lori Sandohl, RN, DSN, CW, OCN; Nancy Toth, RN, BSN; Bonnie Koch, RN, OCN; Carol Ann Peters, RN, MSN; Bruce Nicholson, MD; Diane Erdos, RN, MSN; Sharon Olson, RN, MSN; Irena Rusenas, MS; Eric Pfeiffer, BA; Margaret Davitt, RN, MSN; Susan A. Rokita, RN, MSN; Sandra Frey, RN, OCN; Shirley Faddis, MSN, OCN; Katherine Yoder, RN, OCN; Diane Blum, ACSW; Carolyn Messner, ACSW; Mary Lander, RN; Barbara Robinawitz, PhD; Harold Piety; William Sattazahn, Jr.; Marion Sattazahn; Kenneth Kohler; Timothy Freer; Edward Henry; Marjorie Cassel; and Marion Spangler. We appreciate the help of Barbara Van Horn and Renee Atchison Ziegler of the Institute for the Study of Adult Literacy in editing the manuscript to maximize readability of the chapters.

We also express our appreciation to the following people for their support and suggestions during this project: John Stryker, MD; Frank Davidoff, MD, FACP; Thomas Feagin, MD, FACP; Charles Lewis, MD, FACP; Nick Leasure, MD; David Hufford, PhD; Steven Hulse, MEd; Judy Lyter, RN, BS; Catherine Kleese, RN, OCN; Mary Jo Templin, RN; Janice Mills, RN, MS; Bonnie Bixler, MEd; and Julia Yost.

Administrative support from our host institutions has been invaluable in carrying out this work and is greatly appreciated. These include the Departments of Behavioral Science and Medicine of the Pennsylvania State University College of Medicine; the Department of Clinical and Health Psychology, School of Health Professionals, Allegheny University of Health Professions; the Department of Nursing of Bloomsburg University; and the Johns Hopkins Oncology Center.

While each chapter was reviewed and edited by many persons, certain people played special roles by contributing significantly to the first versions of the chapters and by actively participating in their revisions and final editing. They are:

Dale B. Schelzel, RN, OCN: *Nausea and Vomiting, Tiredness and Fatigue, Vein Conditions (Needle Sticks), Appetite;*

Sandra J. Spoljaric, RN, OCN: *Mouth Conditions, Hair Loss;*

Kathy B. Kambic, RN, OCN: *Diarrhea, Constipation;*

Dale B. Schelzel RN, OCN; Allan Lipton, MD; and Harold A. Harvey, MD: *Fever and Infections, Bleeding;*

Elise M. Givant, RN, OCN; Peter S. Houts, PhD; Allan Lipton, MD; Harold A. Harvey, MD; Matthew J. Loscalzo MSW; and James R. Zabora, MSW, ScD: *Getting Information from Medical Staff;*

Mary A. Simmonds, MD; Georgia Brown, RN, BSN; Bruce Nicholson, MD; and Julia A. Bucher, RN, PhD: *Cancer Pain;*

Sandra J. Spoljaric, RN, OCN; and Mary Lander, RN: *Skin Conditions;*

Carol Nolt, MSW; Matthew J. Loscalzo, MSW; James R. Zabora, MSW, ScD; and Julia A. Bucher, RN, PhD, OCN: *Getting Help from Community Agencies and Volunteer Groups;*

Arthur M. Nezu, PhD; Christine M. Nezu, PhD; Peter S. Houts, PhD; Matthew J. Loscalzo, MSW; James R. Zabora, MSW, ScD; and Eric Pfeiffer, MS: *Anxiety, Depression;*

Julia A. Bucher, RN, PhD: *Coordinating Care from One Treatment Setting to Another, Mobility (Moving Around the House), Sexual Conditions;*

Joan F. Hermann, LSW: *Helping Children Understand;*

Peter S. Houts, PhD; Julia A. Bucher, RN, PhD; Carol D. Nolt, MSW; Glenda M. Trumpower, MSW; Matthew J. Loscalzo, MSW; James R. Zabora, MSW, ScD; and Carole A. Bean: *Understanding Caregiving.*

An important resource for the *Understanding Caregiving* chapter was the Caring Families manual developed by the Family Caregiver Project at the University of North Carolina at Charlotte. The authors of the Caring Families manual were D. D. Fernald, PhD; James R. Cook, PhD; and Catherine A. Gutman, DrPH, RN. Its development was supported by Grant No. 90PD0153 from the Office of Human Development Services of the U.S. Department of Health and Human Services.

Other important sources of information included *Helping People Cope: A Guide for Families Facing Cancer* developed by the Cancer Control Program of the Pennsylvania Department of Health and authored by Joan F. Hermann, ACSW; Sandra L. Wojtkowiak, RN, BSN; Peter S. Houts, PhD; and S. Benham Kahn, MD, as well as many informational booklets and brochures developed and distributed by the American Cancer Society and the National Cancer Institute.

An earlier version of this book was published in 1994 by the American College of Physicians under the title *Home Care Guide for Cancer*. The editors and publishers appreciate the permission given by the American College of Physicians to adapt and update material from the *Home Care Guide for Cancer in the Guide to Caregiving.*

Contents

Preface

Now, more than ever, we are winning the fight against cancer. Scientific and technical advances in cancer medicine have increased the chances of extending life and have even increased the chance of a cure for most types of cancer. Furthermore, there have been important advances in controlling symptoms and side effects of treatment, so that the quality of life of people with cancer can be better now than it ever was in the past.

However, these advances in cancer treatment also have made cancer care more complex. Treatment often includes surgery, radiation therapy, and chemotherapy, as well as other therapies. Frequent tests are often required to monitor the effects of treatment. Cancer treatments often go on for months and then must be resumed if the disease returns. As a result, you (people with cancer, their families, and other caregivers) must be prepared to cope with a wide range of physical, emotional, and social consequences of the disease and treatments for extended periods of time. In addition, as time in the hospital is shortened and more treatments are given in the doctor's office or clinic, you are taking on greater responsibility for managing care at home. You are assuming many responsibilities that, until recently, have been carried out by health professionals. Cancer care professionals now rely on you to monitor medications, manage side effects, and report conditions that require professional intervention.

It is our experience that caregivers and people with cancer can carry out these responsibilities if given clear guidance from health professionals. *Caregiving* provides this guidance. Chapters were written by cancer care professionals with many years of experience and with help from home caregivers and people with cancer. The chapters give the information you need for managing care and preparing for conditions, rather than just responding to crises.

Caregiving also helps you work cooperatively with health professionals. If you follow the guidelines in these chapters, then professional staff know that you are following procedures recommended by cancer care professionals. Furthermore, since the chapters identify when to call for professional help, staff can be assured that if the guidelines are followed, they will be kept informed when certain conditions need their attention.

Peter S. Houts, PhD
Julia A. Bucher, RN, PhD

How to Use This Book

This book consists of five sections: *Cancer Treatments, Managing Care, Emotional Conditions, Physical Conditions,* and *Living with Cancer and Cancer Treatments.*

The *Cancer Treatments* section summarizes the six major types of treatments used to control cancer: surgery, chemotherapy, radiation therapy, biological therapies (which use the immune system to treat cancer), hormone therapy, and bone marrow and peripheral blood stem cell transplants. This is "foundation" information for caregiving. It explains the different treatments, why and when they are used, and the effects they can have on people receiving the treatments. This section also has information about clinical trials and financial considerations.

The *Managing Care* section explains different issues of caregiving, how to help children understand cancer and its course, coordinating care, getting help from community resources, and obtaining information.

The *Emotional Conditions, Physical Conditions,* and *Living with Cancer and Cancer Treatments* sections deal with situations or conditions that may occur when giving care to a person with cancer.

The *Appendix* has a diagram of a typical drug label and an explanation of how to read it accurately. The *Resource Guide* provides programs and services that may be of special interest to those with cancer and caregivers. A *Glossary* of common terms is also included for quick reference.

How to Read the Chapters

We recommend reading the chapters before you start dealing with a situation or condition. Reading the chapters early allows you to develop orderly plans that you can refine as you gain experience. Having plans also gives you a sense of purpose and hope that can help you cope with the stresses of caregiving. By reading a chapter before situations or conditions develop, you will be able to recognize them early, take action before they become severe, and even prevent some problems from happening.

Reread chapters when situations or conditions persist. Chapters contain many ideas and strategies for dealing with caregiving situations or conditions. It can be hard to remember them all. A good strategy is to reread chapters when a situation or condition persists to be sure you are doing everything you can.

A Six-Step Approach to Problem Solving

The best way to be successful in caring for a person with cancer is to understand the problem you need to solve and the desired goal. Some examples of problems you may encounter as a caregiver include a breakdown in communication between yourself and the person with cancer, asking for assistance from others, or serious side effects or conditions as the result of treatment.

There are six steps needed for successful problem solving:

Step 1: Use positive thinking to help solve problems.

Step 2: Understand the situation or condition.

Step 3: Decide if you need professional help.

Step 4: Plan what you will do.

Step 5: Consider obstacles and how to deal with them creatively.

Step 6: Develop, carry out, evaluate, and adjust your plan.

STEP 1: Use positive thinking to help solve problems.

One of the most important things you can do to help the person you are caring for is to have a positive attitude toward solving caregiving problems. At the same time, be realistic about the seriousness of the condition so the person you are helping does not feel that his or her condition is being ignored or belittled.

The day-to-day issues of coping with cancer can seem overwhelming to both of you. However, if you expect to solve those problems, you both will feel in control. One of the best ways to do this is to break situations into manageable pieces and to set reasonable goals that you have a good chance of achieving. Resolving big issues in small steps is an important part of good caregiving.

Expect to succeed. If you believe that you can resolve issues, this will help you to try hard and will increase the likelihood of success. On the other hand, if you expect to fail, you may not try your hardest. If you avoid problems or try not to think about them, there is a good chance the situation will get worse.

Having a positive but realistic attitude will increase your chances of successfully solving caregiving problems.

USE POSITIVE SELF-TALK

Stop and listen to the messages you are saying to yourself. For example, if you are feeling tired because of your caregiving work, you might say to yourself, "I'm always tired and can never do anything I need to get done." This "self message" will make you feel depressed. However, if you say to yourself, "I am feeling tired now, but I'm looking forward to taking time tomorrow to do some things I want to do," you will have made a promise to yourself that will help you feel positive and hopeful.

CONTROL NEGATIVE SELF-TALK

Avoid using words like "should" or "ought," and replace them with "hope" and "try." Instead of saying, "I should invite friends to visit," say, "I will try to invite friends."

Challenge irrational beliefs and overgeneralizations. If you think "I'm a failure," challenge those thoughts. Say, "No, that's wrong, there are times when I have been successful." Then think of a time when you were successful.

QUESTION WORDS SUCH AS "DISASTER" AND "HOPELESS," AND THINK CAREFULLY ABOUT WHAT REALLY HAPPENED

Use positive self-statements such as "I can solve this problem; I don't have to please everyone; I can cope with this; I can reduce my fears; it's normal to feel upset in this situation."

RECOGNIZE THAT PROBLEMS ARE INEVITABLE

Problems are a part of life, and it is normal to have them when you are giving care to someone with a serious illness like cancer.

Ask yourself, "How have my problems changed since I have become a caregiver?" Many problems will be the same as before, others will be worse, but some will be better.

Use your feelings as cues or signals to tell you that a situation needs to be solved. Negative feelings may be a sign that a situation is there. Transform your negative feelings into positive ones by starting to solve the problem that makes you upset.

REALIZE THAT YOU ARE ALREADY AN EFFECTIVE PROBLEM-SOLVER

Dealing with situations that come with caring for someone with cancer takes training and practice. However, you have a head start because you have been dealing with challenges all of your life at home, at work, with friends, and with family. You are also capable of solving caregiving problems. This book will help you to make the best use of the skills that you already have.

STEP 2: Understand the situation or condition.

A well-defined problem is a situation half solved. A good place to start is the *Understanding the Situation or Condition* section featured in each chapter. These sections have information about what causes the situation or condition, who tends to have them and when, and the kinds of things that can be done. You can also ask your doctor, nurse, or social worker for information and recommendations.

GET THE FACTS

You need to know the facts about your special condition. It helps to think of yourself as a detective, investigative reporter, or personal scientist. Don't guess or assume. Separate what might be true from what you know is true. Your job is to know, as clearly as possible, the facts about the condition and to match those facts with information about what can be done about it.

Avoid focusing solely on negative facts. Be sure to acknowledge what went right as well as what went wrong.

Break down the condition into clear, specific details and use objective words. For example, instead of saying, "I'm upset," try, "I feel upset because I don't see my friends anymore." By stating your problem precisely, other people can understand exactly what you mean, and you give yourself a clear goal to work toward.

Separate facts from impressions and assumptions. Try not to say, "The nurse doesn't like me anymore." Instead say, "When I passed her in the hall she didn't notice me." The second way of stating the problem doesn't make any assumptions and shows that there are many possible reasons why she didn't notice you and that she may still like you.

Identify exactly what makes a situation troublesome. It doesn't help to get into a panic and say, "He's getting worse." Instead, try saying, "He feels warm, and I wonder if a fever may be starting." The first statement is too general, but the second statement tells you what to do (that is, take the temperature and read the chapter on fever to decide if you need to call a doctor).

Set realistic goals. A realistic goal is one that you have a reasonable chance of reaching if you try. If you set unrealistic goals for yourself (for example, expecting to do everything you used to do before you started caregiving), you are setting yourself up for failure. By setting goals that you can achieve (such as talking to a friend on the phone instead of having a meal together), you can feel that you have accomplished something.

Understanding the situation or condition and having the facts about them is the foundation you need to carry out an effective and realistic plan. Writing down what is happening often helps people to view facts objectively. Talking to people who have had similar conditions can help you see your own situation more objectively. Ask at the doctor's office, hospital, or your local American Cancer Society office where you can find a support group of people facing similar problems.

STEP 3: Decide if you need professional help.

The first question to ask is whether professional help is needed. For physical conditions, you must get professional help since the health of the person you are caring for depends on it. For emotional and social problems, professionals can give you guidance in developing your plans and, in the case of severe depression or anxiety, they can give specialized counseling or therapy.

The *When To Get Professional Help* section in each chapter tells when to call for help. This can help you decide whether help is needed immediately or if it's something that can wait until office hours. It also details what information to have ready when calling a doctor or nurse, so you get the help you need as fast as possible.

STEP 4: Plan what you will do.

If professional help is not needed at this time (or if help has already been given), there are still things you can do to help manage the problem on your own. This includes things to prevent the problem from getting worse and to reduce discomfort.

The *What You Can Do to Help* section of each chapter lists what other people have found helpful in managing their caregiving problems. Look through these lists to find ideas that may help you. We recommend regularly reviewing the lists of things you can do in this book to be sure you are doing everything you can.

You can also get ideas for what you can do from family, friends who have dealt with similar problems, support groups, and from community service agencies and hospitals. See the chapters *Understanding Caregiving* (pages 32–45) and *Getting Help from Community Agencies and Volunteer Groups* (page 69–77) for ideas on how to make use of these resources.

STEP 5: Consider obstacles and how to deal with them creatively.

Each person is unique, and each problem is unique. Therefore, you will need to be creative in adapting your plans to fit each unique situation.

Most plans will run into obstacles or roadblocks. Overcoming or sidestepping these obstacles will also challenge your creativity. When your plans don't work out as you had hoped, see this as a challenge to your creativity.

The *Possible Obstacles* section in each chapter lists some common obstacles that other family caregivers have had in dealing with the same problem. Use the list as a start, then think of obstacles that could prevent you from dealing with your problem and develop creative solutions.

CREATIVITY IS THE KEY

There are many ways to be creative. Here are some suggestions:

- Talk to someone about the situation or imagine what another person would do. Explaining a problem to someone else helps you to see it more clearly. You can even imagine that you are talking to someone and get help without the person actually being there.

- Improve on something that worked a little bit. Too often we discard ideas that worked a little bit because they weren't completely successful. The fact that it worked a little bit means that there is some part that was working. Try to find out what was good about it, and use that as a basis for a new idea.

- Try a smaller goal. Too often we think we are not successful when, in reality, we are making progress. We are just expecting change too fast. So the creative solution may be to scale down what we hope to accomplish so that it matches what we can accomplish. Another way of saying this is: If at first you don't succeed, try a smaller goal.

- Brainstorm. Make a list of ideas that might be useful. Any ideas you have, no matter how strange or even silly, should be included on the list. Make your list as long as possible. The more ideas you have, the better the chance that one of them will be helpful. Other people can often help you think of ideas that you wouldn't have thought of alone.

  Choose ideas likely to succeed. And, finally, go over the list one more time with a critical eye and choose the ideas that have the best chance of being successful.

STEP 6: Develop, carry out, evaluate, and adjust your plan.

Think about what you and other people need to reach your goal. Involve the person you are caring for as much as possible in both developing and carrying out the plan. It should be his or her plan as well as yours. If others are involved, think about how you will work with them.

The *Carrying Out and Adjusting Your Plan* section of each chapter offers suggestions on how to organize your plan and check on results. It also recommends what to do if your plan is not successful.

Keeping a record or diary of what you did, and the results will help you see what was successful and also give you ideas for dealing with similar problems in the future.

If your plan isn't working, think of obstacles as challenges. Review what you have done and develop a new plan.

Ask yourself if your goal was reasonable. Perhaps you really were making progress, but you were expecting change too fast. If this is the case, change your goal to something more reachable and work toward your larger goal gradually.

Revise your plan and keep on trying! **Always have a plan and don't give up!**

Cancer Treatments

This section explains the different treatments, why they are used, and what to expect before, during, and after receiving them. This information will help you understand what will be happening to the person you are caring for so that you can help the person with cancer get through these experiences.

Use this section as needed; you may not need to read the entire section, only those parts that apply specifically to the person you are helping. For instance, the person you're caring for may initially have surgery and then chemotherapy. So you may want to read only those sections. Later, the person's doctor may recommend hormonal therapy. You then can return to this section to review the information on hormonal therapy so that you know what to expect.

Understand Informed Consent Before Receiving Any Type of Cancer Treatment

Before starting any cancer treatment, the person with cancer should feel comfortable that they understand what has been explained to them about the therapy and that all their questions have been answered. Once this has occurred, the person will provide written permission to receive the therapy. This process of receiving and understanding the information is called informed consent. This permission should be based on the person's understanding of the following:

- the treatment recommended by the doctor or oncologist (a physician who specializes in treating people with cancer)
- how it will be performed and how long it will take
- the potential risks and benefits of the treatment
- what the potential side effects are and how they will be treated
- what other options are available to the person with cancer

The person with cancer should know the answers to these questions before signing a consent form. His or her signature means the person has received this information and that he or she is willing to have treatment.

Surgery

Surgery is the treatment of disease, injury, or disfigurement by means of an operation. It is the oldest form of treatment for cancer and offers the greatest chance for cure for many cancers. About 60 percent of people with cancer will have some type of surgery. This form of treatment is usually recommended to achieve one or more goals.

- **Preventive (or prophylactic) surgery** is performed to remove a growth that is not yet malignant (cancerous) but is likely to become malignant if left untreated.
- **Diagnostic surgery** is used to obtain a tissue sample for lab testing to confirm a diagnosis and identify the specific cancer.
- **Staging surgery** determines the extent of disease and how far it has spread. For example, doctors may perform laparoscopy and laparotomy (described later in this section) to assess organs in the abdomen. Other tests are performed to stage other types of cancer.
- **Curative surgery** is the removal of a tumor when it appears to be localized and there is hope of taking out all of the cancerous tissue.
- **Palliative surgery** is performed as a treatment of complications of advanced disease and is not intended to cure cancer. It is also intended as an effort to correct a condition that is causing discomfort or disability.
- **Supportive surgery** is used to help with other types of treatment, such as the delivery of pain medicine or chemotherapy. For example, a vascular access device (a port) is placed under the skin to give chemotherapy treatments.
- **Restorative (or reconstructive) surgery** is used to restore a person's appearance or restore the function of an organ or body part.

Surgery Can Be Used to Diagnose

- **Biopsy** is a procedure to remove all or part of a tumor for tests. Some types of biopsies involve operations to remove an entire organ. Other types of biopsies may remove tumor samples through a thin needle or endoscope (a flexible lighted tube). These biopsies are sometimes done by surgeons, but also can be performed by other doctors such as radiologists, oncologists, pathologists, or gastroenterologists (see *Glossary*).
- **Fine needle aspiration (FNA) biopsy** uses a very thin needle and an ordinary syringe to withdraw a small amount of tissue from the tumor. The doctor can aim the needle while feeling a suspicious tumor or area near the surface of the body. If the tumor is deep inside the body, the needle can be guided while it is viewed by a computed tomography (CT) scan. The main advantage of FNA is that it does not require a surgical incision (cutting through the skin). The disadvantage is that in some cases this needle cannot remove enough tissue for a definite diagnosis.
- **Excisional or incisional biopsy** is when a surgeon cuts through the skin to remove an entire tumor (excisional) or a small part of a large tumor (incisional). This often can be done with local anesthesia or regional anesthesia (numbing medication). If the tumor is inside the chest or abdomen, general anesthesia is used (the person is asleep).
- **Endoscopy** uses a very flexible tube with a viewing lens or a video camera and a light on the end. If a video camera is used, it is connected to a television set. Both allow the doctor to see any masses in the area. The endoscope can be passed through natural body openings to view suspicious areas in the gastrointestinal tract, genitourinary tract, and the respiratory tract. Endoscopy helps the doctor directly view the cancer mass and take a tissue sample through the endoscope to determine whether cancer is present and, if so, what type it is.
- **Laparoscopy** is similar to endoscopy but is used to examine the contents of the abdomen and remove tissue samples. A tube is passed through a tiny incision in the abdomen. (A similar procedure to view the inside of the lungs is called bronchoscopy.)

- **Laparotomy** is a technique that involves an incision into the abdomen, usually a midline incision from the upper to lower abdomen. This may be done when there is uncertainty about a suspicious area that cannot be diagnosed by less intrusive tests, such as by x-rays. During the laparotomy, a biopsy of a suspicious area can be done and an assessment can be made about the location, size, and spread into surrounding areas. This technique involves general anesthesia in which the person is put to sleep.

Surgery Can Be Used to Treat

There are a variety of types and methods of surgery today because of so many scientific advances. Each of the following types of surgery is explained along with examples of the kinds of cancer they may be used to treat.

- **Laser surgery:** The term "laser" stands for Light Amplification by Stimulated Emission of Radiation. Laser light is a highly focused and powerful beam of light energy that is used in medicine for very precise surgical work, such as repairing a damaged retina in the eye, cutting through tissue (replacing a scalpel), or vaporizing a cancer of the cervix, larynx, or skin. Surgery can be less complicated with laser light. For example, with fiber optics, light can be directed to many parts of the body without making a large incision in the skin.

- **Cryosurgery:** This technique involves the use of liquid nitrogen spray or a very cold probe to freeze and kill abnormal cells. It is sometimes used to treat precancerous conditions such as those affecting the cervix. Cryosurgery is also being studied as a treatment of some cancers such as prostate cancer.

- **Electrosurgery:** This procedure involves the use of a high-frequency electrical current to destroy cells. It is used for some cancers of the skin and mouth.

- **Mohs' surgery:** Also known as microscopically controlled surgery, this is a technique for removing cancerous tissue by shaving off one layer at a time. After each layer is removed, a specially trained dermatologist or pathologist immediately examines the tissue under a microscope. When all the cells look normal, the surgeon stops removing layers of tissue. This technique is used when the extent of cancer is not known or when the maximum amount of healthy skin needs to be preserved (as in cancers around the eye). This is performed under local anesthesia by a specially trained surgeon. Chemosurgery is an older name for this surgery and refers to certain chemicals applied to the tissue before it is removed. The procedure does not involve use of chemotherapy drugs.

The Risks Associated with Surgery

In most situations, the chance that surgery will cause cancer to spread is very small. However, there are a few important exceptions. Doctors who are experienced in taking biopsies of cancers and treating them with surgery are very careful to avoid these situations.

The chances of a needle biopsy causing a cancer to spread are extremely low. In the past, larger needles were used for biopsies and the chances were more significant. Most types of cancers can be safely sampled by an incisional biopsy, but there are a few exceptions. For these types of cancer, doctors may recommend removing the entire tumor if it is likely to be cancerous. In other cases a needle biopsy can be safely used and if that indicates a tumor is cancer, surgery to remove it will follow.

Some types of cancers have the potential to spread into the surgical wound when an incisional biopsy is done. Surgeons doing such a biopsy will be certain that the skin surrounding the biopsy site is in a location that can later be completely removed as part of the follow-up operation to remove the entire cancer.

A Second Opinion Is Invaluable

When a person learns he or she needs any surgical procedure, getting opinions from at least two surgeons is helpful in deciding whether or not to proceed with the operation.

The person's doctor will not mind this extra step. In fact, some insurance companies require a person get a second opinion. Tests may not need to be repeated since the results often can be sent to the second doctor.

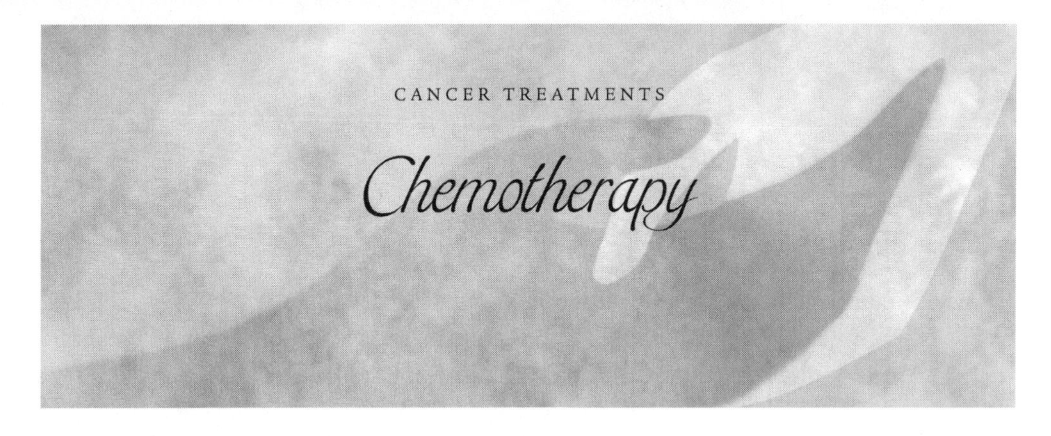

Chemotherapy, the use of medicines, is one of several treatments used to help people with cancer. Depending on the type of cancer and its stage of development, chemotherapy can be used:

- to cure cancer
- to keep cancer from spreading
- to slow cancer's growth
- to kill cancer cells that may have spread to other parts of the body from the original tumor
- to relieve symptoms that may be caused by the cancer

Although a single drug can be used to treat cancer, generally chemotherapy (anticancer) drugs are more powerful when used in combination. Today, about 80 different chemotherapy drugs are used to fight cancer. Combination chemotherapy uses drugs with different actions to kill more cancer cells and reduces the chance that a person will develop a resistance to one particular drug.

Some chemotherapy drugs kill cancer cells so tumors may shrink or even disappear. Other drugs work by stopping cancer from spreading. Each anticancer drug has a different job to do.

Chemotherapy is not new. It has been helping people since the early 1950s. These drugs have been tested repeatedly over the years and have been shown to work.

Sometimes chemotherapy is the only treatment a person receives. More often, chemotherapy is used in addition to surgery and/or radiation therapy. Some people have surgery and chemotherapy. Others have radiation and chemotherapy. Still others have all three types. There are several reasons why chemotherapy may be given in addition to other treatment methods.

- Chemotherapy may be used to shrink a tumor before surgery or radiation therapy is started.

- It may be used after surgery or radiation therapy to help destroy any remaining cancer cells.
- It may be used with other treatments if cancer returns.

When chemotherapy is given following surgery to destroy any cancer cells that may still be present, it is called adjuvant therapy. When chemotherapy is used to shrink a tumor before surgery or radiation therapy, it is called neoadjuvant therapy.

Drug Delivery Methods Vary

Chemotherapy is given in a number of different ways. Depending on the type of cancer and the drug or drugs given, a person may receive chemotherapy these ways:

- By mouth in a pill, capsule, or liquid form. The person with cancer will swallow the drug, just like many other medications. This method usually is more convenient and may be less expensive since the drugs can be taken at home. If the person is taking drugs orally at home, it is important to make sure he or she takes the exact dosage that has been prescribed.
- By injection using a needle into a muscle, under the skin, or directly into a cancerous area in the skin.
- On the skin. The medication will be applied onto the surface of the skin.
- Into a vein. There are several ways this can be done. The person will get the drug through a thin needle inserted into a vein, usually on the hand or forearm. The drug may be given over a few minutes—which is called an intravenous (IV) push—or as an infusion that can last 30 minutes or a few hours. Continuous infusions are sometimes necessary and usually last one to several days.

Intravenous infusions are also given by means of a catheter, a thin tube that is placed into a large vein in the body and remains there as long as it is needed. This type of catheter is known as a central venous catheter. Sometimes, a central venous catheter is attached to a port, a small plastic or metal container placed surgically under the skin, usually in the chest.

Catheters may also be placed into the spinal canal, abdominal cavity, bladder, or liver. The doctor or nurse may use specific terms when talking about certain types of catheters. These include:

- intrathecal catheters, which are used to deliver drugs into the spinal fluid;
- intracavitary catheters, which are placed in the abdomen, pelvis, or chest;
- intra-arterial catheters, which deliver chemotherapy drugs directly into an artery to treat a single area (such as the liver, or an arm or leg). This method limits exposure of the drug to a specific part of the body.

If a catheter is used, another device—a pump—may also be used to help control how much drug enters the body over time. External pumps remain outside the body. Many are very small—about the size of a portable CD player. Some are portable and on wheels. These allow a person to move around while the pump is in use. Other external pumps are not portable and may restrict activity. Another type of pump is internal. Internal pumps are placed surgically inside the body, usually right under the skin. They contain a small reservoir (storage area) that delivers the drugs into the catheter that goes to the vein or specific target site.

Treatment Schedules Vary

Cancer affects everyone differently, so types and amounts of chemotherapy vary for different people. It may be given once a day, once a week, or even once a month, depending on the individual and his or her type of cancer.

Whatever schedule the doctor prescribes, it is very important to encourage the person to stay with it. Otherwise, the anticancer drugs might not have their desired effect. If a treatment session or a dose of medication is missed, contact the doctor for instructions about what to do.

Sometimes, the doctor may delay a treatment based on the results of certain blood tests. The doctor will let the person know what to do during this time and when it's okay to start treatment sessions again.

Other Medicines May Interfere

Some medicines may interfere with the effects of chemotherapy. To avoid any complications, you can help the person you're caring for by writing a list for the doctor of all medications being taken, including prescriptions, herbal remedies, vitamins, and any over-the-counter medications (such as aspirin, laxatives, cold pills, pain relievers, and so on). Include the name of each drug, the dose, how often it's being taken, and the reason for taking it.

After reviewing the list, the doctor will tell the person with cancer if he or she should stop taking any of these medications before starting chemotherapy. After treatments begin, be sure to check with the doctor before the person begins taking any new medicines or stops taking any of those on the original list.

How It Feels to Get Chemotherapy

Taking chemotherapy by mouth or by injection generally feels the same as taking other medications by these methods. Having an IV injection usually feels like having blood drawn for a blood test. Some people feel a coolness or other unusual sensation in the area of the injection when the IV is started. Any feelings of discomfort or pain should be reported, whether they occur before, during, or after treatments.

Many people have little or no trouble having the IV needle in their hand or lower arm. However, if a person has a hard time for any reason, or if it becomes difficult to insert the needle into a vein for each treatment, it may be possible to use a central venous catheter or port. This avoids repeated insertion of the needle into the vein.

Central venous catheters and ports cause no pain or discomfort if they are properly placed and cared for, although a person usually is aware that they are there. It is important to report any pain or discomfort with a catheter or port to the doctor or nurse.

Many people are able to continue working while they are being treated with anticancer drugs. It may be possible to schedule treatments late in the day or right before the weekend, so they interfere with work as little as possible.

Other chapters in this book provide further details about coping with the side effects associated with chemotherapy and about taking care of veins and receiving chemotherapy.

How to Determine If Chemotherapy Is Working

Doctors and nurses use several methods to measure how well chemotherapy treatments are working. People with cancer can expect to have frequent physical examinations, blood tests, scans, and X-rays and should not hesitate to ask about the test results and what they mean, especially in terms of progress.

While tests and examinations can tell a lot about how chemotherapy is working, side effects tell very little. Sometimes people think that if they don't have side effects, the drugs aren't working, or that, if they do have side effects, the drugs are not working well. However, side effects vary so much from person to person, and from drug to drug, that having them or not having them usually isn't a sign of whether the treatment is effective.

Chemotherapy and the Family

Cancer isn't contagious, so the person you're caring for can go on being close to family and friends. Depending on how the person's body reacts to anticancer drugs, people may not notice he or she is on chemotherapy at all. If he or she does get unpleasant side effects, you, the family, and friends can do things to help. When someone asks "How can I help?", have a few suggestions ready. The person with cancer may not want to eat much, and family members can take turns cooking foods that help him or her feel like eating. The person with cancer might get tired after each treatment and need extra rest. Family members can do little jobs for the person with cancer until he or she feels better.

Encourage the person you're caring for to take his or her family's help with a smile, which makes their loved ones feel better. Because they care so much, family and friends might be nervous about chemotherapy. You should encourage the person with cancer to be honest about how he or she feels. There will be times when the people closest to the person with cancer may also feel tired or blue, and you can help by reminding them how much you value their aid.

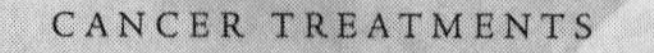

Radiation Therapy

Radiation therapy is the treatment of cancer and other diseases with high-energy particles or waves, such as x-rays, gamma rays, electrons, and protons, to destroy or damage cancer cells.

Radiation therapy is one of the most common treatments for cancer and is used in more than half of all cancer cases. It is the primary treatment for some types of cancer, such as:

- certain nonmelanoma skin cancers;
- some head and neck cancers;
- early stage Hodgkin's disease and non-Hodgkin's lymphomas;
- some cancers of the lung, breast, cervix, prostate, testes, bladder, thyroid, and brain.

Radiation therapy is also known as radiotherapy, x-ray therapy, and irradiation. Radiation deposits energy that injures or destroys cells in the area being treated (the "target tissue") by damaging their genetic material, making it impossible for these cells to continue to grow.

All cells, cancerous and healthy, grow and divide. However, cancer cells grow and divide more rapidly than many of the normal cells around them. Radiation therapy uses special equipment to deliver high doses of radiation to cancerous tumors, killing or damaging them so that they cannot grow, multiply, or spread. Although normal cells in the field of treatment will be affected by radiation, most appear to recover fully from the effects of the treatment. Unlike chemotherapy, which exposes the entire body to cancer-fighting chemicals, radiation therapy affects only the tumor and the surrounding area.

For some kinds of cancer, radiation alone can cure the cancer. It is more likely, however, to be used with other types of treatment. Radiation can also reduce pressure, bleeding, pain, or other symptoms caused by advanced cancer or large tumors.

The radiation used in radiation therapy can come from a variety of sources. The doctor may choose to use x-rays, an electron beam, or gamma rays. Choosing which type of radiation to use depends on what type of cancer the person has and on how deep into the body the doctor wants the radiation to penetrate. High-energy radiation is used to treat many types of cancer. Low-energy x-rays are used to treat some kinds of skin diseases.

Many people become free of cancer after receiving radiation treatments alone or in combination with surgery, chemotherapy, or biologic therapy.

Treatment from a Team of Specialists

A doctor who has had special training in using radiation to treat disease—called a radiation oncologist—will prescribe the type and amount of treatment that best suits the person's needs.

The radiation oncologist works closely with other doctors and also heads a highly trained health care team. Other members of the radiation therapy team may include the following:

- The radiation physicist makes sure that the equipment is working properly and ensures the machines deliver the right dose of radiation.
- The dosimetrist helps carry out a doctor's treatment plan by calculating the number of treatments and how long each treatment should last.
- The radiation therapy nurse provides nursing care and helps the person with cancer learn about treatment and how to manage side effects.
- The radiation technician operates the radiation equipment and positions the person receiving treatment.

A dietitian, physical therapist, social worker, and other health care professionals also may be needed to help people receive radiation therapy and cope with cancer.

Two Types of Radiation Therapy

Radiation therapy is given in two forms: external and internal. Some people receive both types of therapy.

External radiation (or external beam radiation) requires a machine that directs high-energy rays at the cancer and some normal surrounding tissue. Most people receive external radiation therapy during outpatient visits to a hospital or treatment center.

Internal radiation therapy (or brachytherapy) places the source of the high-energy rays as close as possible to the cancer cells so that fewer normal cells are exposed to radiation. By using internal radiation therapy, the doctor can give a higher total dose of radiation in a shorter time than is possible with external treatment.

Instead of using a large radiation machine, the radioactive material is placed directly into (or as close as possible to) the affected area. Some of the radioactive substances used for internal radiation treatment include radium, cesium, iridium, iodine, phosphorus, and palladium.

Internal radiation therapy often is used for cancers of the head and neck, breast, uterus, thyroid, cervix, and prostate.

Pretreatment and Planning Are Key

After a physical examination and a review of the person's medical history, the radiation oncologist may need to do some special planning to pinpoint the treatment area. In a process called simulation, the person with cancer will be asked to lie very still on a table while the radiation therapist uses a special x-ray machine to define the exact place on the body where the treatment will be aimed. There may be more than one site on the body. Simulation may take from a half hour to about two hours. It marks the exact site for radiation to be pointed.

The radiation therapist often will mark the treatment area on the skin with tiny dots of colored, semipermanent ink to outline the treatment area. Care should be taken when bathing to not wash off these marks until all the treatment is over. If they start to fade, the therapist should be told and he or she will darken them so that they can be seen easily.

Using the information from the simulation, other tests, and medical background, the doctor will meet with the radiation physicist and the dosimetrist. The doctor then decides how much radiation is needed, how it will be delivered, and how many treatments will be administered. This process often takes several days before radiation treatment is started.

Length of Treatment Plans Vary

Radiation therapy usually is given five days a week for up to eight weeks. When radiation is used for palliative care (to relieve symptoms), the course of treatment lasts for two to three weeks. Both of these types of schedules, which use small amounts of daily radiation, rather than a few large doses, help protect normal body tissues in the treatment area. Weekend rest breaks allow normal cells to recover. The total dose of radiation and the number of treatments received will depend on the size and location of the person's cancer, the type of tumor, his or her general health, and any other treatments being provided.

How It Feels to Get Radiation Therapy

External Radiation

External radiation treatments are painless. The experience is just like having a regular x-ray taken. The actual treatment takes only a few minutes; however, each session can last 15 to 30 minutes because of the time required to set up the equipment and correctly position the person getting treatment.

Depending on the treatment area, the person may need to get undressed and wear a hospital gown. In the treatment room, the radiation therapist will use the marks on the skin to locate the treatment area. Then the person will sit in a special chair or lie down on a treatment table under the radiation machine.

The radiation therapist may put special shields (or blocks) between the machine and certain parts of the person's body to help protect normal tissues and organs. There might also be plastic or plaster forms to help the person stay in exactly the right place. The person will need to remain very still during the treatment so that the radiation reaches only the area where it's needed and the same area is treated each time.

Once positioned correctly, the radiation therapist will leave the treatment room before the machine is turned on. The person getting treatment will be watched on a television screen or through a window in a nearby control room and can communicate with the therapists at any time.

The machines used for radiation treatments are very large, and they make noises as they move around to aim at the treatment area from different angles. Their size and motion may be frightening at first. Remember that the machines are being moved and controlled by the radiation therapist. They are checked constantly to be sure they're working right.

A person getting treatment will not see or hear the radiation. In case he or she feels ill or very uncomfortable during the treatment, the therapist should be told and the machine can be stopped at any time.

Internal Radiation

When internal radiation is given, the radiation is placed in the affected tissue, usually in small tubes or containers. These implants may be temporary or permanent. Internal radiation may also be given in capsule form by mouth or by injecting a solution of radioactive substance into the bloodstream or a body cavity.

For most types of implants, the person will need to be in the hospital and have general or local anesthesia while the doctor places the container for the radioactive material in the body.

To get the radiation as close as possible to the cancer, doctors may use implants of radioactive material sealed in wires, seeds, capsules, or needles. The type of implant and the method of placing it depend on the size and location of the cancer. Implants may be put right into the tumor, in special applicators inside a body cavity, on the surface of a tumor, or in the area where the tumor has been removed.

The radioactive substance in the implant may transmit rays outside the body. While receiving implant therapy, the hospital may require the person with cancer to stay in a private room. Although nurses and other caregivers will not be able to spend a long time in the person's room, they will provide all necessary care. In most cases, the urine and stool will contain no radioactivity. However, either one may contain some radioactive material if unsealed internal radiation therapy was used.

There will also be limits on visitors while the implant is in place. Most hospitals do not let children younger than 18 or pregnant women visit people who have an implant. Visitors should sit at least six feet from the person's bed and stay for only a short time each day (10 to 30 minutes). Visitors should ask the nurse for specific instructions before entering the hospital room.

The total amount of time that an implant is left in place depends on the dose (amount) of radioactivity with which the person is treated. The implant may have a low dose rate and be left in place for several days, or a high dose rate and removed after a few minutes. Generally, low dose rate implants are left in place from one to seven days.

For some cancer sites, the implant may be left in place permanently. If the implant is permanent, the person with cancer may need to stay in a hospital room away from other people in the hospital for a few days while the radiation is most active. The implant will lose energy each day, so by the time the person is ready to go home, the radiation will be much weaker.

High dose rate implants allow a person to be treated within a few minutes in inpatient or outpatient clinics. A very powerful radioactive source travels by remote control through tubes, or catheters, to the tumor. The radioactivity remains at the tumor for only a few minutes. In some cases, several remote treatments may be required. Sometimes the catheter stays in place between treatments and sometimes it is removed, depending on the person's condition.

Follow-Up Care

Once the course of radiation therapy is finished, it is important to have regular examinations to check the results of treatment. The radiation oncologist will want to see the person being treated at least once after treatment ends. The doctor who referred the person for radiation therapy will schedule follow-up visits as needed. Follow-up care, in addition to checking the results of treatment, might also include more cancer treatment, rehabilitation, and counseling.

Most people with cancer return to the radiation oncologist for regular follow-up visits. Others are referred back to their original doctor, to a surgeon, or to a medical oncologist.

Just as every person with cancer is different, follow-up care varies. The person may find he or she needs extra rest while healthy tissues are rebuilding. The person may need some time to test his or her strength, little by little, and a full schedule may not be advised right away.

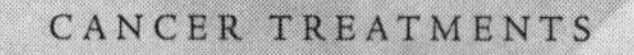

Biological Therapies

Biological therapy (sometimes called immunotherapy, biotherapy, or biological response modifier therapy) is a promising new addition to the family of cancer treatments. Biological therapies use the body's immune system to fight cancer or to repair normal cells that may be damaged by some cancer treatments.

The body has a natural ability to protect itself against diseases, including cancer. The immune system, a complex network of cells and organs that work together to defend the body against attacks by "foreign" invaders, is one of the body's main defenses against disease.

Researchers have found that the immune system may recognize the difference between healthy cells and cancer cells in the body and eliminate those that become cancerous. Cancer may develop when the immune system breaks down or is overwhelmed. Biological therapies are designed to repair, stimulate, or enhance the immune system's natural anticancer function.

Immune system cells and proteins called antibodies, which are part of the immune system, work against cancer and other diseases by creating an immune response against foreign invaders (antigens). This immune response is unique because antibodies are specifically programmed to recognize and defend against certain antigens. Antibodies respond by latching on to, or binding with, antigens, fitting together much the way a key fits a lock.

Biological response modifiers (BRMs) change the interaction between the body's immune defenses and cancer, improving the body's ability to fight the disease. BRMs are substances that occur naturally in the body. Scientists now can make BRMs in the laboratory. They can play many roles in cancer treatment, including slowing or stopping tumor cell growth and acting to help healthy cells, particularly immune cells, control cancer. BRMs may be used to:

- enhance a person's immune system to fight cancer cell growth;
- eliminate, regulate, or suppress body responses that permit cancer growth;
- make cancer cells easier to destroy by the immune response;
- change the growth patterns of cancer cells so they act more like healthy cells;
- block or reverse the process that changes a normal cell or a pre-cancerous cell into a cancerous cell;
- repair normal cells damaged by other forms of cancer treatment, such as chemotherapy or radiation;
- prevent a cancer cell from spreading to other sites in the body.

How Biologic Therapies Are Administered

Most biologic therapies can be done on an outpatient basis. Biologic therapies are given in one of two ways:

- By injection with a needle into a muscle, under the skin, or directly into a cancerous area in the skin.
- Into a vein. The person will get the drug through a thin needle inserted into a vein, usually on the hand or forearm. The drug may be given over a few minutes—called an IV push—or as an infusion which can last several hours.

Treatment schedules vary and it's important to follow the program developed by the physician.

Hormone Therapy

Hormones are naturally occurring products in the body. Hormonal therapy is used to prevent the growth, spread, or recurrence of cancer. Hormone therapy can block the body's natural hormones from reaching any remaining cancer cells. Estrogens are used in the treatment of prostate cancer and breast cancer. Corticosteroids are used to treat many different kinds of cancer.

If lab tests show that a tumor depends on estrogen or progesterone hormones to grow, it will be described as estrogen-receptor-positive or progesterone-receptor-positive in the lab report, as in breast cancer. This means that any remaining cancer cells may continue to grow when these hormones are present in the body.

The basic types of hormone treatments used for people who have cancer are:

- **Corticosteroids (steroids)** are produced by a small gland called the adrenal gland.
- **Estrogens** are female hormones produced by the ovaries.
- **Antiestrogens** are often used to treat cancers in which estrogen promotes growth of cancer, such as breast cancers. They can be used for adjuvant therapy (see page 21) or for treating advanced breast cancer.
- **Progestins** are other hormones produced in the ovaries.
- **Androgens** are male hormones produced by the testes.

- **Luteinizing hormone-releasing hormone (LHRH) analogs** are drugs that decrease the amount of testosterone produced by a man's testicles. LHRH analogs are injected either monthly or every three months at the doctor's office or at the oncology center. These drugs can lower the level of testosterone as effectively as surgical removal of the testicles.
- **Antiandrogens** are drugs that block the body's ability to use androgens. Anti-androgens often are used in combination with orchiectomy or LHRH analogs. This combination is called total androgen blockade. Recent studies indicate that combination therapy may be more effective than LHRH analogs or orchiectomy alone.
- **Diethylstilbestrol (DES)**, a drug chemically related to the female hormone estrogen, was once the main form of hormonal therapy for men with prostate cancer. Because of its side effects (which include increased risk of heart disease), it has been mostly replaced by LHRH analogs and antiandrogens.
- **Intermittent hormonal therapy** is a treatment option for men with prostate cancer. Nearly all prostate cancers treated with hormonal therapy eventually become resistant to this treatment over a period of months or years. Some doctors believe that continuous exposure to hormonal drugs might provide some resistance and recommend intermittent treatment with these drugs as an alternative.
- **Adjuvant hormonal therapy** is treatment used in addition to the main (usually surgical) treatment. Adjuvant hormonal therapy is often used to treat breast cancer, and is an option for some men with prostate cancer.
- **Aromatase inhibitors** are drugs that stop estrogen production by blocking an enzyme responsible for producing small amounts of that hormone in women after menopause. Aromatase inhibitors can be used as an adjuvant therapy for early breast cancer or for treating advanced breast cancer.

Bone Marrow and Peripheral Blood Stem Cell Transplants

Bone marrow and peripheral blood stem cell transplants are used to treat people with cancer when a person's bone marrow—spongy tissue found in the center of bones that produces blood cells—is damaged and cannot make the red blood cells, white blood cells, or platelets the body needs. These types of treatments are also used when high doses of chemotherapy and radiation therapy are needed.

Bone marrow transplantation (BMT) replaces diseased or damaged bone marrow with new, functioning bone marrow. Peripheral blood stem cell transplantation (PBSCT) involves the removal of stem cells–immature blood cells–from blood prior to chemotherapy. The cells are returned to the person after chemotherapy treatment to enrich the damaged and weakened blood.

BMT and PBSCT are used because high doses of chemotherapy and radiation therapy can severely damage or destroy a person's bone marrow so that he or she is no longer able to produce needed blood cells.

Destroying the marrow may be a part of treatment for diseases that affect the bone marrow (such as leukemia), or it may simply be a side effect of treatment for cancers that affect other parts of the body. In any case, BMT and PBSCT allow stem cells that were damaged by treatment to be replaced with healthy stem cells that can produce the blood cells the person needs.

Bone Marrow Transplants

There are three basic types of BMT: autologous, allogeneic, and syngeneic. The source of bone marrow used determines the type of transplant.

- **Autologous BMT** means the person with cancer is the donor. Bone marrow is taken from the patient, frozen until needed, and then returned (transplanted) after the person receives high doses of chemotherapy, radiation therapy, or both. Autologous BMT is used to treat forms of cancer that do not involve bone marrow (such as ovarian cancer, lymphoma, breast cancer, and brain tumors) or diseases that affect the bone marrow but are in remission.

  Autologous BMT is the most common type of BMT. Because the donor and recipient are the same person, some of the complications associated with allogeneic transplants are avoided.

- **Allogeneic BMT** involves replacing bone marrow with new, healthy bone marrow from a donor. The best donor is someone whose tissue type matches that of the person who is being treated. Usually the donor is a family member, such as a brother or sister. However, for people who don't have a family member with matching bone marrow, it is sometimes possible to find a donor in the general population through a bone marrow registry.

- **Syngeneic BMT** occurs when the donor is an identical twin. This is an ideal situation because the donor and recipient have identical tissue types. However, this sort of transplant is rare (less than one percent) because relatively few people have identical twins.

Peripheral Blood Stem Cell Transplants

Peripheral blood stem cell transplants, with or without bone marrow transplantation, is being studied for its usefulness in treating some of the same diseases. People who have cancer cells in their bone marrow or who do not have enough stem cells in their marrow may be considered for PBSCT.

All blood cells develop from immature cells called stem cells. Most stem cells are found in the bone marrow, although some, called peripheral blood stem cells, circulate in blood vessels throughout the body.

In PBSCT, the stem cells usually come from the person with cancer. Stem cells are removed from the his or her circulating blood before treatment and then returned after treatment.

Finding Donors

The increase in transplants using marrow from unrelated donors has been possible in part through the existence of large bone marrow registries, such as the National Marrow Donor Program (NMDP) and the American Bone Marrow Donor Registry (ABMDR).

The NMDP coordinates searches among donor and transplant centers throughout the United States and other countries. The ABMDR is a privately funded registry of a large number of potential marrow donors. A smaller agency, the Caitlin Raymond International Registry, can access more than 3.8 million international donor records.

Transplant Pretreatment Procedures

Before the actual transplantation, the person undergoes several days of laboratory and diagnostic tests. Doctors check the person's general medical condition, looking for signs of infection or damage to organs from previous treatment. A dental examination is generally recommended to make sure the mouth is as healthy as possible before treatment begins because treatment will likely cause it to become sensitive and easily infected.

An IV catheter usually is surgically placed in one of the large veins in the chest. The catheter is used for drawing blood samples; for giving blood or blood products, antibiotics, other drugs, and nutritional support; and for transplanting the new marrow.

Catheters generally can remain in place for many months. (Before they leave the hospital, people are taught how to care for the catheter at home.)

Procedures for Allogeneic or Syngeneic Donors

Donors normally stay in the hospital for one or two nights because most receive general anesthesia, which puts them to sleep. The use of newer anesthetics has made bone marrow donation possible as an outpatient procedure at some centers.

Bone marrow is removed from the pelvic (hip) bones and, in rare cases, from the sternum (breastbone) as well. Generally, four to eight small cuts are made in the pelvic area, and a large needle is inserted through these cuts to draw the marrow out of the bones.

Procedures for Autologous (Self) Transplantation

In autologous transplantation, people with cancer receive their own marrow or peripheral stem cells. For autologous transplantation to be successful, the person's marrow must be relatively free of disease when it is harvested (removed). In some people, autologous transplantation works best because the cancer does not involve the bone marrow. In people who have leukemia and lymphomas, initial treatments to make the cancer disappear are necessary before bone marrow harvesting.

Procedures for PBSCT

Peripheral stem cells are harvested in a less complicated process called apheresis or leukapheresis. In this procedure, blood is removed through an IV catheter or through a large vein in the arm and is run through a machine that removes stem cells. The rest of the blood is returned to the person with cancer. This usually takes two to four hours and is repeated an average of six times. There usually is no need for hospitalization or anesthesia.

Conditioning Is an Important Step before Transplantation

Conditioning—treatment with high-dose chemotherapy with or without radiation therapy—is important for the success of the transplantation. Its primary purpose is to destroy cancer cells throughout the body more effectively than may be possible through conventional treatment. In addition, cells in the marrow are destroyed, creating space for the new marrow. In people undergoing allogeneic transplantation, conditioning serves a third purpose: because it destroys the cells of the immune system, it reduces the risk that the recipient will reject the new marrow.

Follow-Up Care

Most people stay in the hospital for one to two months after bone marrow transplantation. This is necessary to monitor success and to treat any potential complications, such as infections. The use of growth factors can shorten the time many people must spend in the hospital. Growth factors are substances produced normally by the body that speed up the regrowth of blood cells.

Many people need a full year to recover physically and psychologically from transplantation. Even after that period, life may not return to the way it was before the illness: medication may be necessary indefinitely, and the person's lifestyle may have to be changed to help prevent fatigue, avoid infectious diseases, and cope with the long-term effects of treatment.

Family caregivers are also affected by the lomg-term effort of caring for people undergoing bone marrow transplantation. Home health visiting nurses can assist the family greatly during recovery.

How to Determine If the Transplant Is Working

A successful transplantation (engraftment) usually takes between two and four weeks. The first sign that the engraftment is taking place is an increase in the white blood cell count. Until engraftment occurs, people are very susceptible to infections (because of the lack of white blood cells) and bleeding (because of a lack of platelets).

To reduce the risk of infection during this period, contact with other people is limited to the BMT team and just a few visitors. No children are allowed to visit.

The transplant is considered a failure when bone marrow function does not return or when it is lost after a period of recovery. Unsuccessful transplantations usually result from one of two reasons: either the recipient's body rejects the donated marrow, or the transplanted stem cells fail to grow and produce new blood cells.

Clinical Trials

Clinical trials are carefully designed research studies that test promising new cancer treatments. Some doctors may suggest that a person with cancer join a clinical trial for cancer treatment, or he or she may want to bring up this option with their doctor. People who take part in research may be the first to benefit from improved treatment methods. These people can also make an important contribution to medical care because the results of the studies may help many others. Clinical trial participants typically receive the best care available and are monitored carefully by a number of specialists who are aware of privacy concerns and care about the participants' well-being. Patients in Phase III clinical trials usually receive either the best standard treatment available or a new therapy with the potential to be even more effective. Participation in clinical trials is completely voluntary and people are free to withdraw at any time.

There are many ways to find a clinical trial. The best place to start is with the person's oncologist. Many trials are carried out in university hospitals or cancer centers and research institutes, but some are available in community hospitals.

To learn more about clinical trials, call the American Cancer Society at (800) ACS-2345, or the National Cancer Institute's Cancer Information Service at (800) 4-CANCER.

Paying for Treatments

The cost of treatment varies with the kinds and doses of drugs used, how long and how often they are given, and whether they are taken at home, in a clinic or office, or in the hospital. Most health insurance policies (including Medicare Part B, which helps pay for doctors' bills and many other medical services) cover at least part of the cost of many kinds of these treatments.

In an effort to reduce their costs, some private insurance companies are deciding not to pay for the use of some drugs or therapies, even if they are effective cancer therapies. Before beginning treatment, find out whether your insurance company or Medicare will pay for the therapy.

Teamwork with the doctor and office staff is important. Be sure to let them know if payment has been denied. They can consult with the insurer and help answer any questions the insurer may have. They can also consult with the company that makes the drug or drugs that are being taken. Often, these companies can provide information or other services that will help get payment.

In some states, Medicaid (which makes health care services available for people with financial need) may help pay for certain treatments. Contact the office that handles social services in your city or county to find out whether the person with cancer is eligible for Medicaid and whether the therapy is a covered expense.

If help is needed to pay for treatments, contact the hospital's social service office. They may be able to direct you to other sources of help in your area. The resource guide at the end of this book provides contact information for many organizations.

If as a caregiver, you are a family member or are responsible for the family finances, you may want to provide assistance in collecting information about paying medical or hospital expenses. It is important that the person with cancer deals with financial problems early—before they become crises. If you are responsible or partially responsible for the family finances, you may want to sit down with the person with cancer to discuss these issues, or work on them yourself. Don't put it off. The earlier you start working on this problem, the easier it will be to solve. If you talk to the people to whom money is owed before it becomes a crisis, they are usually willing to work with you. The following is a checklist of things that you can do to help solve this problem:

- **Collect the facts.** First, collect information about current expenses and those expected in the future, as well as about all of the financial resources. You will need this information to decide what help is needed and what criteria have been met to qualify for assistance. If you decide to ask for help, you will be asked to provide this information.

- **Figure out the medical expenses.**

  1. *How much is owed for medical expenses?* This is often difficult to determine, especially with the confusing way that many hospitals and other health care organizations send their bills. Most hospitals and doctors' offices have someone on their staff who understands the billing forms. These people can quickly go through a stack of bills and determine exactly what is owed at that time.

  2. *What future expenses are anticipated?*

  3. *Approximately how much has been paid out so far for medical care during this illness?* Keep track of the medical expenses that are not covered by insurance since these may be deductible from income taxes. Copies of bills and cancelled checks will help demonstrate the need for financial assistance.

- **Figure out the financial resources.**

  1. *What kind of medical expenses does the insurance company cover?* This is important information to have even before the bills arrive. It helps you to estimate what the expenses will be. Ask the insurance agent or the workplace health insurance representative.

  2. *How much money is in the savings account?*

  3. *What assets are there (house, property, stocks)?*

  4. *What is the total income of the household?* Household income is the total income of everyone living in the same household with the person with cancer. This information is often used to calculate eligibility for financial assistance.

- **Investigate spacing out paying bills or paying in installments.** Contact the financial counselor or the business credit office in the hospital. They can help you set up a monthly payment plan. Some hospitals, doctors, and pharmacies submit bills to the insurance company and bill for what the insurance company won't pay. This saves people from paying the bills and then waiting for reimbursement from the insurance company. Ask the hospital or doctor's office if they will do this.

- **Investigate borrowing money.** Banks and other organizations that lend money will want to know about the financial situation and about money that is expected to be received in the future. Collect this information before you talk to them. Shop around for the best terms and the most reasonable interest.

- **Apply for financial assistance.** Many people are eligible for financial assistance and do not know it. Social workers are usually the best source of information about how to get help with medical expenses and who qualifies for help. Most hospitals employ social workers and if the person you are caring for is a patient there, you can make an appointment with a social worker. However, if the hospital is far from your home, the hospital social worker may not be familiar with resources in your community.

  People on disability, veterans, and people receiving vocational rehabilitation services often qualify for financial assistance for cancer treatments. Ask the social worker to check that you are receiving your benefits.

  Other sources of financial help include the American Red Cross, county boards of assistance, and United Way agencies. Sometimes they will help with past expenses as well as future expenses. These agencies are listed in the white and blue pages of your telephone book. Hospital social workers will often help you find and apply for help from community organizations. You can either call the social work department yourself or ask the doctor or nurse to refer you to them.

  Family, friends, and community groups can often help people in financial need due to illness. Some community groups have funds to help group members, but others, especially religious groups, have funds to help anyone in need. Talk to members of community organizations and churches about your needs.

Managing Care

This section will help you manage the care of a person with cancer. *Understanding Caregiving* summarizes ways of being an effective caregiver, and *Helping Children Understand* may give you some insight on dealing with younger members of the family affected by cancer. Often it is necessary to transfer or relocate the person with cancer to various facilities, such as a rehabilitation center or a nursing home. *Coordinating Care from One Treatment Setting to Another* addresses these issues. *Getting Help from Community Agencies and Volunteer Groups* informs caregivers about accessing resources in the community and *Getting Information from Medical Staff* provides information about getting medical information.

The information in this section is about caring for the person with cancer. It fits most situations, but yours may be different. If the doctor or nurse tells you to do something else, follow what they say. If you think there may be a medical emergency, see the *When to Get Professional Help* section of each chapter.

This section explains situations faced by many caregivers and people with cancer. Encourage the person with cancer to read this information, and then you can work together as a team.

MANAGING CARE

Understanding Caregiving

Understanding the Situation

Caregivers are problem solvers

Caregiving involves solving problems. You have been solving problems throughout your life. The only difference now is that many of the challenges that come with cancer are new to you and to the person you are helping. The chapters in this part of the book will help both of you through the new challenges.

While the information in these chapters will help, you and the person with cancer are the ones who will actually solve the problems. You decide what actions to take. You adjust the plans to meet your special situations. You carry out the plans. And you monitor how well the plans are working and make changes as needed. You also develop new plans on your own to deal with situations that are not in this workbook. The six problem-solving steps discussed in the beginning of this book will help you to do this.

Family caregivers are members of a team

The family caregiver is a team player—working with the person with cancer, working with other family and friends, and working with medical staff to solve problems.

The person with cancer is central to the team. The person with cancer should participate in his or her own care and should be involved in all problem-solving discussions that affect him or her. Success requires his or her participation and agreement.

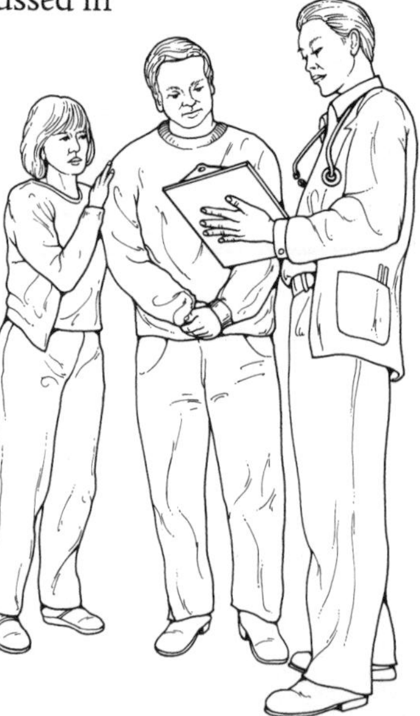

Health care professionals are also key members of the team. Caregivers work with health professionals to ensure the care given at home is consistent with the best medical practices. Since health professionals played a key role in writing this book, you can be sure that if you are following these instructions, you are doing what they would recommend. Health professionals are also a valuable source of information and advice for dealing with problems that are not discussed in this book.

Family members and friends who share in caregiving are also important team members. In addition to helping in practical ways, family members and friends can give encouragement and emotional support, and they can share their experiences and knowledge from dealing with similar problems in their lives.

Work to have a positive attitude toward caregiving

Emphasize the positive parts of caregiving. Some caregivers see their work as helping someone they care deeply about. Many feel that caregiving has enriched their lives. Others see it as a challenge and want to do the best job they can. Some see caregiving as a way of showing appreciation for the love and care they have received themselves, and others see caregiving as spiritually enriching.

Caregiving can have important benefits. Caring for a person with cancer at home can give you a sense of satisfaction and confidence and can show you inner strengths that you didn't realize you had. Caregiving can draw families together and can help people feel closer to the person who needs care.

You can also use caregiving to open doors to new friends and relationships by talking to other people who have faced the same problems. This could include meeting people in a support group, talking to health professionals who showed understanding and concern, and relying on family members who have grown distant but who are drawn together because of a difficult situation.

Caregivers need to take care of themselves

Helping someone who is going through cancer treatments can be difficult and stressful. The more you care for your own needs for rest, food, enjoyment, and relaxation, the better you will be able to help the person you are caring for. There is a section later in this chapter titled "Taking care of your own needs and feelings" with ideas for how to organize positive experiences for yourself and how to notice and remember the good things that are happening in your caregiving. These ideas are important because they will help you to be a better caregiver.

Your goals for caregiving are to:

- be an effective team member working with health professionals, family, and friends
- involve the person you are caring for in your caregiving plans as much as possible
- be an advocate for the person with cancer to be sure that he or she gets needed information and services
- take care of your own needs so that you have the emotional and physical strength to be an effective caregiver

When to Get Professional Help

Ask for help from health professionals, a member of the clergy, or other professionals if any of the following conditions exist:

- **You are not able to carry out your caregiving responsibilities, and the needs of the person whom you care for are not being met.** Social workers, clergy, nurses, and physicians can help you get the help you need so the person with cancer gets needed help and services.

- **You are experiencing severe anxiety or depression.** It is normal to feel upset and stressed when caring for someone at home for a long period of time. Read the chapters on anxiety (pages 88–99) and depression (pages 100–113) for a list of symptoms that indicate if professional help is needed.

  Getting help for anxiety or depression is just like getting help for physical problems. Asking for help does not mean you are "crazy." It means that you are wise and even courageous. Professionals such as social workers, counselors, clergy, psychologists, and psychiatrists are skilled and experienced in helping emotionally upset people. Your family doctor can also be helpful in assessing how severe your symptoms are and in recommending a professional to help you.

- **Communication between you and the person with cancer has broken down or has become painful or difficult.** The stresses that come with cancer—physical, psychological, financial, and emotional—can interfere with your ability to communicate with the person you are caring for. Get professional help if anxiety and stress levels have risen to where you aren't able to talk openly with the person with cancer about important issues.
- **Your relationship with the person with cancer is clouded by a history of abuse or addiction.** Caregivers who have suffered verbal, mental, physical, or sexual abuse from the persons they are caring for, or where alcohol or drug addiction has affected relationships, are likely to have serious problems in caregiving. They already have strong and deep-seated feelings, usually built up over many years. This situation calls for professional help from the start.

What You Can Do to Help

Working and communicating effectively with the person with cancer

This is your most important job. It can also be the most challenging. The person you are caring for is dealing with the physical effects of the disease and treatments as well as with the psychological and social challenges of living with cancer. This may make it difficult for him or her to participate in the plans. Nonetheless, your job is to involve the person you are caring for as much as possible in making decisions and carrying out the plans.

Help the person with cancer deal with the diagnosis emotionally and live as normal a life as possible. Some people with cancer try to deal with upsetting news by pretending that it didn't happen. This can be harmful, however, if they do things that make the illness worse, such as avoiding treatment or doing activities that are physically harmful.

Support the efforts of the person with cancer to live as normal a life as possible. However, if he or she is pretending that nothing is wrong, you need to be clear in your own mind about what is really happening so he or she does not do things that could be harmful.

Create a climate that encourages sharing feelings and supports his or her efforts to share. Talk about important or sensitive topics in a time and place that's calm and favorable to open communication—not in the midst of a crisis or an argument. If your time for talking about problems in your family is around the dinner table, that's the time to do it. Think about when you have had important and constructive talks in the past. Strive to recreate that setting.

Communicate your availability. One of the most important messages you can communicate is "If you want to discuss this issue, I'm willing to listen and talk." However, leave the timing up to him or her. To the greatest extent possible, the person with cancer should make decisions on what feelings to share and when, how, and with whom to share them. By not pressing the issue, you allow the person to retain control over part of his or her life at a time when many issues and decisions are beyond control.

Understand that men and women often communicate in different ways, and make allowances for those differences. Women sometimes express their feelings more openly than men in our society. If you're a male caregiver and the person with cancer is a woman, be aware when she shares feelings. You may find yourself giving advice when she just wants someone to listen and be understanding. If you're a female caregiver and the person with cancer is a man, be aware that he may express his feelings differently than you would. Pay special attention when he talks about things that are important to him. It may be helpful to openly discuss differences in how men and women express feelings and how they like to be supported.

Be realistic and flexible about what you hope to communicate or agree on. People with cancer want to share many things, but they may not share them all with just one person. Let the person talk about whatever he or she wants with whomever he or she wants. It's OK if the person isn't telling you everything, as long as he or she is telling somebody. Also, remember that a person has spent a lifetime developing a communication style, and that won't change overnight.

Sharing doesn't always mean talking. The person with cancer may feel more comfortable writing about his or her feelings or expressing them through an activity. He or she may express feelings in other nonverbal ways, such as by making gestures or expressions, touching, or just asking that you be present. Also, sharing someone's silence can be a wonderful thing and a privilege. Sometimes caregivers just need to respect the person's right to be alone.

Disagreeing on important issues

Remember that you don't have to agree. Two people aren't always at the same place at the same time, and there's no simple answer to many problems—especially if they are long-standing.

Explain your needs openly. Sometimes you may need to ask the person with cancer to do something to make your life easier or your caregiving responsibilities more manageable. Keep in mind that conflict resolution doesn't always mean everybody is happy. On some issues you'll have to give in, and on others you'll ask the other person to give in.

Suggest a trial run or time limit. If you want the person with cancer to try something (such as a new bed or schedule) and he or she is resisting, ask to try it for a limited time, like a week, and then evaluate the situation. This avoids making the person feel locked into a decision. If the person resists writing a will or power of attorney, ask if he or she will at least discuss it.

Choose your battles carefully. Ask yourself, "What's really important here? Am I being stubborn because I need to win an argument?" You can save energy by skipping the minor conflicts and using your energy and influence on issues that really count.

Let the person with cancer make decisions. Taking away a person's ability to make decisions can undermine feelings of control, which interferes with the ability to deal with other aspects of this stressful illness. A good example is when adult children living some distance away from a person with cancer want to move him or her into a nursing home. Although moving the person with cancer to a nursing home may make the adult children feel better, this may not be what the person with cancer wants. If the person with cancer understands the consequences (for example, no one may be around to help if he or she falls), he or she has the right to make that decision.

Taking care of your own needs and feelings

You need to be at your best to do the best job of caregiving. Therefore, be aware of your own needs as well as those of the person you are helping. Set limits on what you can reasonably expect of yourself. Take time off to care for yourself and your needs and ask for help before stress builds up.

Schedule positive experiences for yourself. There are three types of positive experiences that you need for good mental health:

1. enjoyable activities with other people (having lunch with a friend, attending a support group meeting)
2. activities that give you a sense of accomplishment (cooking a special meal, exercising, finishing a project)
3. activities that just make you feel good or relaxed (watching a funny movie, playing with a pet, taking a walk)

Plan these activities regularly. And when you are away from caregiving try to be completely away from it. Don't think about it or talk about it. This is your time to "recharge your batteries" by being involved in something different than caregiving.

Pay attention to positive experiences. Make an effort to notice and talk about pleasant experiences as they happen during the day. Watch the news or take time to read the morning paper. Set aside time during the day, like a meal, when neither of you will discuss the illness.

Getting help from others

Don't try to do everything yourself. If you do, caregiving can wear you out, increase your stress, and interfere with your ability to give good care at home. Consult the chapter *Getting Help from Community Agencies and Volunteer Groups* (pages 69–77) to learn about services such as support groups and home health agencies that are available in your community. The *Resource Guide* at the end of this book will also help you find assistance in getting help. Make arrangements for fill-in help from family members and friends.

Sometimes caregivers withdraw from family and friends, especially as caregiving gets more difficult. They don't feel like talking about their problems, or they're so busy that they don't find time to be with others. However, caregivers need to have a social life. It is a fact that caregivers who have support from other people become less depressed and overwhelmed about the responsibilities of caregiving. If you isolate yourself from others you lose the stimulation from other people and you lose the suggestions and help that others can give.

Reach out to others and involve them in your life and in your caregiving. This is also important for the person you are caring for. To do this you need to make visiting rewarding for the visitor so he or she wants to come again. Here are some things you can do:

- Make a list of people who can give companionship and support to you and the person you are caring for. Don't worry about how far away these people live, how busy they are, how long since you've talked to them, or even how well you know them. Make as long a list as you can to give you the most choices.
- Go down your list and, for each person, think what you could do to make a visit (or a phone call) pleasant and enjoyable. Use these ideas when you invite them and when they visit or call. This way they will want to come again and you will feel good about asking them to return.
- Have a list of ways visitors can help in case they offer or if you feel comfortable asking. Make your list specific so the person understands exactly what is needed. They will be able to budget their own time and be prepared to give the help you need.

____

____

____

____

____

____

____

____

____

____

____

____

Dealing with strong feelings that you may have

It is natural to have strong feelings when helping someone with a serious illness like cancer. The following is a list of strong feelings that caregivers can have and strategies for dealing with them if they become severe.

FEELING OVERWHELMED

Sometimes problems from caregiving and from other parts of your life build up to the point where you feel overwhelmed. If this happens, here are some things to think about.

Try not to make important decisions when you are upset. Sometimes you have to make decisions immediately, but often you don't. Ask the doctor, nurse, or social worker how long before a particular decision has to be made.

Take time to sort things out. It is important to take some time to let your thinking become clear again. Different people need different amounts of time for this to happen. Give yourself enough time to become more emotionally stable so that you can make plans and decisions with a clear mind and a peaceful spirit.

Talk over important problems with others who have been levelheaded and helpful in the past. If you are feeling upset or discouraged, ask a friend, neighbor, or family member to help. They can bring a calmer perspective to the situation as well as new ideas and help in dealing with the problems you are facing.

ANGER

There are plenty of reasons for someone to become angry while caring for an ill person. Some people feel angry because their lives have been turned upside down by taking on caregiving responsibilities. The person they are caring for may, at times, be demanding and irritable. Sometimes people are angry because they are used to fixing things, and cancer and its problems are not easily fixed. Also, friends, family members, or professionals may not be as helpful or understanding as you would like.

These feelings are normal! It is all right to feel this way at times. It is what you do with your feelings that is important. The best way to deal with angry feelings is to recognize them, accept them, and find some way to express them appropriately. If you don't deal with your anger, it can get in the way of almost everything you do.

Here are some ways that other caregivers have dealt with their anger:

Try to see the situation from the other person's point of view and understand why he or she acted that way. Recognize that other people are under stress too, and some people are better than others in dealing with stressful situations.

Express your anger in an appropriate way before it gets worse. If you wait, your anger may lead to actions and words you may later regret. Anger that is out of control can cloud your judgment. Talk to the people involved and explain why you feel the way you do–but in a way that doesn't make them angry. Or talk to someone who is not involved about why you feel angry. Explaining to another person why you feel angry helps you to understand the reasons for your anger and why you reacted the way you did.

Find safe ways to express your anger. This can include such things as beating on a pillow, yelling out loud in a car or in a closed room, or doing some vigorous exercise. Try writing down why you're so mad. Keep a diary and write down your feelings.

Get away from the situation for a while. Try to cool off before you go back and deal with what made you angry.

GUILT

Many people caring for a person with cancer feel guilty at some time during the illness. They may feel guilty because they think they did something to cause the cancer or because they feel they should have recognized the cancer sooner. They may feel guilty for not doing a better job of giving care or for taking time for their own needs. They may feel guilty because they are angry or upset with the person who has cancer. And caregivers may feel guilty because they are well, and the person they care deeply about is sick.

Although feeling guilty is understandable, it can interfere with doing the best possible job of caregiving. Guilt makes you think only about what you did wrong. In fact, the caregiver may have done absolutely nothing wrong, yet he or she still feels guilty. Most problems have many causes and what you did is only part of the reason for the problem. For example, if you feel anger toward the person you are caring for, this may be partly because of what he or she did as well as what you did. Caregiving is a two-way street.

Here are some ways other caregivers have dealt with feelings of guilt:

Talk to other people who have gone through similar experiences about what happened and how they felt. It is often easier to see a situation objectively when it happens to someone else, and this can give you perspective on your own problems.

Don't expect yourself to be perfect. Expecting perfection in yourself can cause guilt to be a regular part of your life. It is helpful to remember that you are human, and therefore you will make mistakes from time to time.

Don't dwell on mistakes. Accept mistakes and get beyond them as best you can. The chapter on depression has useful ideas for controlling negative thinking by replacing it with positive, creative thoughts (see pages 107–111).

FEAR

You may become afraid when someone you care for deeply has a serious illness. You do not know what is in store for him or her or for yourself, and you may be fearful that you won't be able to handle what happens.

Here are some things other caregivers have done to deal with their fears:

Learn as much as possible about what is happening and what may happen in the future. This can reduce fear of the unknown and help you to be realistic so that you can prepare for the future. Talk with health professionals and with other people who have cared for someone with cancer to see if you are exaggerating the risks.

Read the chapter on anxiety (pages 88–99). The ideas and techniques in that chapter can be used by you as well as by the person with cancer.

Talk to someone about your fears. It often helps to explain your fears to an understanding person. This helps you to think through the reasons for your feelings. Also, talking to a sympathetic person will show you that other people understand and appreciate how you feel.

LOSS AND SORROW

Caring for someone you love but who has changed because of cancer can make you sad. Memories of how healthy and alert the person used to be may make you sad. You may also feel unhappy because of losing "normal" things you did before this illness and because of plans you had for your future that may not be fulfilled. Here are some things you can do about these feelings:

Talk about your feelings of loss with other people who have had similar experiences. People who have cared for a person with cancer will usually understand how you feel. Support groups are one way to find people who have had similar experiences and who can understand and appreciate your feelings.

Read the chapter on depression (pages 100–113). Feelings of loss are often a part of feeling depressed. The ideas and techniques in the depression chapter can help you to manage or prevent depression.

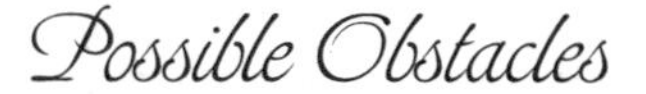

Think about what could prevent you from being an effective caregiver.

Here are some situations that have been difficult for other caregivers:

"He doesn't want to talk about feelings."

He is the best judge of that. Your job is to make sure the opportunities are there to share when he decides it is right.

"What if she talks about things that I don't want to hear?"

Even if what you hear hurts you, it may be helpful for her to express it. You don't have to solve anything. You're being helpful if you just listen.

"He won't follow my advice."

Try to understand how important it is for him to retain some control. You may know what's best for him, but realize that your main job is support. Your job is not to make the decision for him. If you have a dominant personality or have been the one to make decisions in your family, you may have to give some of that control back to the person you are caring for.

"I'm swamped with problems, so I don't have time to take care of my needs."

This is the most common reason caregivers become exhausted. They become preoccupied with problems and don't pay attention to themselves. You will be a better caregiver in the long run if you take the time, especially when stress is high, to do things that you enjoy and that relax you.

"If I don't do it, it won't get done."

Sort out things that really need to be done versus what you would like to see done. It's OK to let some things, like housework, slide a bit when you take on new responsibilities. You can also ask family and friends for help instead of trying to do everything yourself.

"I hate to ask other people to help me."

There are two ways around this problem. You can get together socially with people who could help and let them volunteer, or you could have someone else ask for help for you. Read the section *Getting Help from Others* (pages 38–39) for ideas about how to make others' visits pleasant and rewarding. This will make it more likely that they will want to help.

"My father doesn't want other people to help us."

Suggest trying to get help for just a short time, and then you can talk over how it worked. Also, explain that you are the one who needs help, not him.

Think of other obstacles that could interfere with carrying out your plan

What additional roadblocks could get in the way of your being an effective caregiver? For example, will the person you are caring for cooperate? How will you explain your needs to other people? Do you have the time and energy to carry out these responsibilities?

Develop plans for getting around these roadblocks using the six problem-solving steps discussed in the first section of this book (see pages xi–xvi).

Carrying Out and Adjusting Your Plan

Start using the ideas in this chapter now. Don't wait until you feel overwhelmed. It is easier to develop good caregiving habits and attitudes early on before problems get out of hand.

Set reasonable goals for yourself. It takes time and experience to improve your caregiving skills. Be patient with yourself. You always want to do better but also recognize that you are basically doing a good job.

Checking on results

Every week or so take time to think about how you are doing as a caregiver. Think back over your caregiver experiences and notice how much you have learned and how much better you are now than when you started. Reread this chapter periodically to see if there are ideas here that can be of help.

If your plan doesn't work...

Be realistic about what you can expect of yourself. Don't expect perfection. Everyone makes mistakes. Be kind to yourself.

If you cannot do the things that are essential for the person you are caring for, talk to a social worker, nurse, or doctor about getting the help you need.

If you become so upset that it interferes with your ability to do what needs to be done, review the section *When to Get Professional Help* (pages 34–35) in this chapter for suggestions about how to find professionals who can help you deal with the stresses of caregiving.

Helping Children Understand

Understanding the Situation

A diagnosis of cancer creates changes and stress for all members of the family. At the same time it can also unite a family and be a time for family members to help and support each other—to solve the many problems they face together. With support and help from adults, children can learn and grow emotionally through this difficult experience.

A child's security is built around routines and stability. Changes that the child has no control over threaten the child's security. When an adult member of the household is diagnosed with cancer, there are often changes in the routines, relationships, and experiences the child is accustomed to. Changes may occur in the person with cancer's appearance and energy levels, in the distribution of household duties, the amount of attention children receive, and the people who are in the home. Children need to understand why these changes happen, and, as much as possible, they need stable routines.

For children, it is important that adults be honest in order to foster trust. Children are observant and sensitive to changes in the people they care about. Without you telling them, they can figure out that something is wrong. They will notice facial expressions and tone of voice. They will overhear snatches of conversations. Without clear and honest communication, children will often create their own explanations for the changes, and their imagination may paint a picture worse than reality.

Sometimes parents are so overwhelmed by the diagnosis, the decisions that must be made, and the treatments that they may overlook the child's feelings. Because many families haven't experienced this level of stress before, it may be helpful to talk to a doctor, a counselor, or a member of the clergy to help work out problems. Getting professional help when it is needed is not a sign of weakness and is nothing to be embarrassed about.

Problems that can occur when children are not informed:

- Children may put their own interpretation on the information. They may worry about getting cancer themselves, fear that no one will take care of them, or feel guilty—believing they did something to cause the illness.
- Not talking about cancer may suggest that it is too terrible a topic to discuss and increase the child's fear of the disease.
- Children may find out the truth from someone else and feel betrayed that you didn't tell them.
- Fears of the unknown or that grown-ups are hiding something can aggravate other problems children may already be having due to changes in their family life—such as sleep or appetite problems, difficulties in school, withdrawal, irritability, or fighting.

Reasons why it is important to tell a child that an adult in the household has cancer:

- Children have an excellent ability to adapt to the truth. Even upsetting truths can be helpful in relieving worry and anxiety about what is happening.
- Children can learn they are important and needed by their family during times of stress.
- Children can help the person with cancer and give support during this difficult time. This may even help children cope with stress and changes.

Therefore, telling a child clearly and honestly about cancer can be very important.

Guidelines for talking with a child about cancer

- Be a careful listener and ask the child what he or she wants to know.
- Answer his or her questions clearly and honestly. Especially with younger children, it is useful to give only the information the child asks for—using words matched to his or her age level.
- Be aware that children have special needs at certain ages. Preschoolers, for example, may feel overwhelmed or confused with too much information while older children may want to

learn as much as they can about cancer. (See the section *Age-Group Issues* on pages 60–61 for a discussion of how children in different age groups respond to cancer and suggestions for how to address their concerns.)

Breaking the news

Children don't need to know everything about every test—especially if they're younger. However, if an adult family member is diagnosed with cancer, tell the children soon—certainly before treatment begins. Try to find a quiet place where you can talk without interruptions. If there are children of very different ages, you may want to talk with each of them separately or by age group. Keep in mind the brief attention span of younger children. Remember that, especially for young children, feeling secure is important. So don't forget to say, "We'll always love you, and we'll always be sure that you are cared for."

At the very least, tell a young child the following:

- **The diagnosis.** For example:

  "Mom is sick with a disease called breast cancer."

- **What treatments are expected, how they will affect the person, and how they might affect the young child.** For example:

  "I'm going to have surgery, which means removing the part of me that's not healthy. I won't be able to pick you up or hug you for a while, but I want you to sit next to me real close."

  "Grandpa is going to have strong medicine which will make his hair fall out for a while. He'll look different for a while, but he'll still be Grandpa."

  "Dad is going to have less energy for a while. He'll need to rest more. We'll need to pick quiet times to do things together."

- **The prognosis (chances of a cure).** You may choose to share this information only in response to direct questions from your child. If the prognosis is clearly very good, by all means, reassure the child. If the prognosis is less clear, focus on reassuring him or her that someone will be always there. For example:

  "The doctors expect the treatment to get rid of the disease so I will live to be very old."

  "Dad is taking very strong medicine to get rid of the disease, and we hope it will make him better."

At the end of this chapter is a summary of children's expectations and needs for ages 2 to 5, 6 to 12, and adolescents, as well as what you can do to help children in each of these age groups cope with your illness.

Coping with cancer is an opportunity for strengthening family bonds. Families often draw closer as they work together to overcome the stress and uncertainties of the illness.

Your goals are to:

- tell children clearly what is going on and how it will affect the person with cancer and the rest of the family
- listen to what children say about the illness and about what is going on in their lives
- anticipate problems children may have and try to deal with them early, before they become severe
- get help from doctors, nurses, social workers, clergy, or counselors, if needed, in talking with your children about cancer
- get help for a child if his or her behavior suggests serious and prolonged distress
- strive to draw the family closer together rather than allowing this problem to drive you apart

When to Get Professional Help

If you find you can't discuss the issue openly or at all, consider seeking help from an outside source. This might be a school guidance counselor, the child's teacher, hospital or clinic staff, or a cancer support group. One step many families take, even if they don't have difficulty talking about the disease, is to get some early counseling. You may find this helpful in heading off children's fears and anxieties. Again, people who might help include professional counselors, doctors or other medical staff members, hospital or clinic social workers, or members of the clergy.

Symptoms to look for

It is normal for children to change their behaviors upon hearing disturbing news or when living in a home where the routines have been changed by cancer. However, if the behaviors are disruptive for the child and others and last more than a week or two, it is time to seek professional help. Here are some ways you can tell if children are having trouble adjusting to the fact that someone important in their lives has cancer:

- **New or more frequent negative or disruptive behavior.**
- **Sleep disturbance lasting for more than a few days.**
- **Lack of normal appetite.**
- **Physical complaints such as chest pains or stomach pains that persist without clear medical diagnosis.**
- **Isolation or withdrawal that lasts and deepens.**
- **Increasing problems at school, or skipping school.**
- **Loss of interest in what were previously a child's normal activities, hobbies, or sports.**
- **Extreme perfectionism and fear of making mistakes.**
- **Displays of rituals such as frequent hand-washing.**
- **Constant checking for reassurance, despite the presence of a supportive family.**

- **Making suicidal statements.**
- **Another, less common trait to watch for is children who normally behave well suddenly becoming almost perfect**—that is, compliant, quiet, not expressing any feelings, and perhaps isolated. This may also include children not wanting to leave their parents' sides.

To sum up, be on the lookout for any major change in a child's pattern of behavior that is disruptive and lasts over a period of time.

Getting a counselor

The logical place to start looking for help is at the center where cancer treatments are received. Clinics and hospitals often offer support for people with cancer and their families. If help is not available at your treatment center, check the mental health listings in your phone book.

Try to find someone with knowledge about children's reactions at varying ages and developmental levels—it could be a pediatrician, a child psychologist or psychiatrist, a social worker specializing in child and family issues, a school guidance counselor, or a youth pastor.

Here are examples of what you might say when calling:

"My wife was diagnosed with cancer. Between her visits for radiation therapy and my trying to hold down two jobs, things have been hectic at home. Now our 13-year-old son seems to be picking fights at school and not doing his homework. He has gotten detention three times in the last week, and now he's quit the soccer team even though he's their best player. Can I find someone to talk to him, or all of us?"

or

"I was diagnosed with cancer last month. I can't seem to find the right words to tell my nine-year-old daughter about my illness. Every time I start to do it, I chicken out and just can't go through with it. I'm so afraid I'll upset her. My husband is no help, he's just as scared as I am. I need to talk to somebody with some experience in telling children about cancer."

What You Can Do to Help

Helping the child communicate

Almost everything revolves around communication. Keep the lines of communication open between adults and children.

Even if what children say is upsetting, you should continue to encourage them to share openly. Talk to them about changes that are happening as a result of the illness. Often children find it difficult to share their feelings. If so, your goal should be to help the child say, "Yes, this scares me." You may need to say, "Other kids have feelings like this, and it's OK to feel afraid or angry–it's important to share feelings." Sometimes it helps just to recognize that problems are going on in the family and talk about it.

Talking about a child's fear that a beloved adult may die is an especially sensitive topic. Keep in mind that if a child asks about the person dying, he or she may really be asking something else, such as "Will my family stay together if Mommy dies, and if not, what happens to me?" Children often communicate things indirectly, and it may be up to you to open the lines of communication and feelings.

Here are some "communication problem" signs to look for:

- Some children may not want to be separate from an adult and may cling, out of a sense of fear. If this happens, it may be important to talk about feelings of fear.
- Some children avoid feelings by being silly and acting goofy. Such behavior may be a cue that the child is having difficulty facing his or her feelings.
- Some children stay away from the person with cancer because they are afraid he or she will die. If this happens, talk about the importance of getting through this together, even though it is scary.

Try a variety of ways to help children express their feelings:

Encourage younger children to express their feelings through art. Younger children can be encouraged to draw a picture of their feelings. Emotions can be given names and assigned colors; for example, red can represent being angry, yellow can be happy, blue can be sad, and black can be scared. Ask the child to color a circle that shows how much he or she is feeling angry, happy, sad, scared, and so on.

Consider a "feelings bag" with younger school-aged children to help them talk about their feelings. They are beginning to understand the differences between feelings they show and those they keep inside. A paper grocery bag can become a "feelings bag." On the outside, the child can draw or glue pictures that represent feelings that others see. On the inside of the bag, the child can place pictures that he or she is less comfortable sharing with others.

Consider play-acting and role-playing to help learn about children's thoughts and fears. This can also help children express feelings to others. Try switching roles. Ask the child to pretend to be the person with cancer while you take turns as the doctor, the child, or other people who are involved. If older children are worried about how to talk to peers, volunteer to play the friend while he or she practices how to tell the friend about the illness.

Use storytelling with younger school-aged children as a way to talk about fears and clear up misunderstandings. Rather than reading a bedtime story, suggest that you make up a story together. You can begin, creating an imaginary family similar to your own. Once the story is under way, it is the child's turn to continue the story. You and the child can weave the story together, with you providing support and solutions for problems the child identifies through the story.

Encourage older children or teenagers to talk openly. He or she can also become a "cancer explorer" and learn as much as possible about the disease. Adolescents may find emotional help from attending a support group to hear how others are coping with the same issues. Some treatment centers conduct groups specifically for teenagers. Other activities that may help are keeping a diary or writing a story about the family.

Make a conscious effort to be available to the children during this illness. This is because it is natural for adults to focus on the illness and the person's problems. Therefore, establishing a time (daily or weekly) to spend with children will go a long way toward keeping communication open. This time should be free of interruptions or TV, when you can just ask "How are your doing?" or "How has your day been?" It is important to talk about the child's feelings related to cancer issues as well as about the other things going on in his or her life.

Plan how the person with cancer will communicate with the children when he or she is not at home. Things you can do include talking on the phone, sending notes, e-mailing, and making tape-recorded or videotaped messages.

Avoid trying to protect children by not sharing your feelings such as anger, fear, or worries. This may have a negative impact. It may communicate to children that such feelings are unacceptable or abnormal. They may then feel guilty when they have these feelings. A better approach is to share your feelings and how you coped with those feelings. You may tell the child, for example, "I feel very angry that this has happened to us. Sometimes at night I pound my pillow to let the anger out." Or you might say, "Mom was feeling very scared about her treatments, but the doctors and nurses have helped us see the treatments as the strong medicine she needs to get rid of the disease."

Avoid discussing aspects of treatment that are especially scary to children. If, for example, a child is frightened by needles, think about what you'll say when you describe the treatment and minimize what you say about the injections. It is a natural tendency to describe in great detail experiences that are new or difficult. It is better to save those descriptions for the adults who are better able to understand and give you support.

Humor can go a long way toward defusing tensions. Allowing children to laugh and kid around about the situation can lighten the emotional load. For example, some people who have a prosthesis give it a name.

Let children help

Suggest things children can do to help around the house. This will differ among age groups, but everybody can do something to help. Even a two-year-old can give Mommy a hug, and teenagers can help with adult chores. Whatever the task, each child should feel that he or she is contributing to help the family get through this crisis. This helps to give the child a sense of control and participation.

Plan for change

Sit down as a family and discuss some of the changes that may occur. Changes can be very stressful for children. However, changes are less scary if they are expected. This way it is not such a surprise to children when the changes happen. They will know in advance that things will change and part of their role in the family is to help cope with these changes.

Look for opportunities to create rituals and to continue old ones. Rituals can provide stability in the children's lives during this difficult period. These should be pleasant activities that the child can count on, which require minimal effort on the part of the adults. It might be a weekly movie night with popcorn or carry-out dinner, or a weekly overnight at grandma's or a neighbor's. It could be a phone call from the person with cancer every morning during periods of separation.

Include older children in the treatment experience. Bring older school-aged children along to one of the appointments. Doctors and nurses can answer questions the child may have. This will also allow the child to see the hospital or clinic as a friendly and supportive environment, rather than a "dreadful place where people do mean things." If the person with cancer is going to be hospitalized, children should be prepared for what they will see, hear, and smell during hospital visits.

Continue to use rules of discipline and rewards

Continue to set limits on negative behaviors. Discipline can be difficult to enforce when children act up or behave badly as a way of coping with the stresses of a family illness. However, a breakdown in rules can convince children that things are really wrong and thereby add to their feelings of insecurity. Tell children that you love them but will not accept destructive or bad behavior.

Consistently reward good behaviors

Whenever possible, use rewards rather than punishments to guide and manage a child's behavior. Displace a bad behavior by rewarding good behavior that takes its place. Consistency in both rewards and punishments can help the child to feel secure and that his or her world is under control.

Examples of good behaviors are:

- sharing feelings in positive ways
- helping other family members
- cooperation
- being responsible for schoolwork and household chores
- showing consideration and care for you

Special issues for adolescent daughters of mothers with breast cancer

Adolescence is often a time when communication between mothers and daughters is strained. When a mother is diagnosed with breast cancer, many issues can add to that strain. Mothers may ask more assistance from adolescent daughters. Daughters may be very uncomfortable talking about issues related to breasts, as they are undergoing breast development.

Both mother and daughter may have concerns about the daughter's risk of breast cancer due to the mother's diagnosis. Doctors are gaining a much better understanding of breast cancer risk within families. Chances are her risk is only slightly increased from that of other women and that standard screening is what is appropriate. Make sure she is instructed in breast self-examination as she nears the end of adolescence. If the doctor thinks your family history suggests a genetic breast cancer, you may want to look for a clinic that specializes in breast cancer risk assessment. If your doctor is not aware of this resource, contact the American Cancer Society at (800) ACS-2345 or the National Cancer Institute's Cancer Information Service at (800) 4-CANCER.

Possible Obstacles

Here are some obstacles other parents have faced:

"My mother-in-law has given up on me and talks about me as if death is just a matter of time. I can see that my son is taking this in and getting more and more worried."

A good response to your son's grandmother would be, "Please don't think that everyone who has cancer is going to die," and explain to her what you've told your children. You might write a brief letter that says tactfully but frankly, "This is how we're handling it. This is what we want our kids to know. We ask you to respect what we're saying. Let us handle this, and please don't conflict with our message."

You might also arrange for your child to talk to the doctor. Tell the child, for example, that Grandma doesn't know all the information.

TV programs or videotapes about cancer can be helpful. If you think your child would benefit from seeing them, make sure you watch them with your child, so you can explain what they mean and why you wanted the child to see them.

"Megan overheard us discussing how strapped we are for finances with all of the medical bills we're getting. She's started to think we may be losing our house."

When children overhear talk about money worries, they tend to think the worst—that they're not going to have any food or a home. This also applies to discussions about who will take care of your child. You may be talking about arranging for someone to be with your children tomorrow afternoon when you go for a treatment, but the child may misunderstand and think you're planning a caretaker for after death. Discussions about the logistics of arranging child care can also lead a young child to feel abandoned, unwanted, and unloved.

Reassure your children that you love them, and they don't need to worry about whether they'll be cared for. Be very conscious of what you're saying in front of your children or in places where they can overhear. If your house is small or a child's bedroom is right over the dining room where you sit and talk, find another place to talk.

"What if I break down and cry when we tell my child about their Dad's cancer? What if I don't handle all of this perfectly?"

It is OK for kids to see that their parents have feelings. And even if you do lose control and break down, you're still the best people to talk with your child.

"What about the other kids at school? How will they react to my child when they learn her mother has cancer?"

Children's friends and schoolmates can be very supportive or they can be destructive. They can spread rumors, and they can tell your child, "Well, Joey's mother died, so your mother will, too." Your job is to tell your child: "This is what we know, this is what the doctors have told us, and this is what we've read on this." Tell your children that some friends might say things that are different than what you've said. Emphasize that you will always tell them the truth and their friends don't have all of the facts.

In addition, you can try involving teachers, guidance counselors, or a Sunday school teacher. You can ask them to encourage the child's peers to be supportive. Sometimes children say cruel or thoughtless things merely because they lack experience—nobody has ever told them how to be a supportive friend to a child whose mother has cancer.

If your child is an adolescent, you might ask if it is OK with him or her if you answer their peers directly if they ask questions.

"I'm so stretched between my job, taking my wife to clinic appointments, and running to the pharmacy to get her medicine that it seems that my son and I are like ships passing in the night. As soon as I get back from the doctor's office, Sean is leaving for baseball practice. When he gets home, I'm pooped and ready for bed."

The demands of daily living can drain the energy of a family caregiver as well as a person with cancer. Make sure that once a day or once a week, you do something together as a family and that you talk together as a family. It is important to establish one time that won't be interrupted.

Think of other obstacles that could interfere with carrying out your plan

What additional roadblocks could get in the way of doing the things recommended in this chapter? For example, will the person with cancer cooperate? Will other people help? How will you explain your needs to medical staff? Do you have the time and energy to carry out the plan?

Develop plans for getting around these roadblocks using the six problem-solving steps discussed in the first section of this book.

Carrying Out and Adjusting Your Plan

Checking on results

A weekly check-in with each child is a good idea, just to ask: How are you doing? Are you having any problems in school?

Try to anticipate problems. For school issues, periodically talk with your child's teachers and others who interact with your child to make them aware of the situation and to keep alert for major changes in behavior or mood.

One way you can check on results is to ask whether the child is able to continue with normal daily routines. For example, the daily routine of a four-year old might be saying goodbye to Mom and going to nursery school and playing. If your child is in sixth grade, he or she needs to be able to go to school, do assignments, and interact with friends. Children need to be able to pursue the "work" of their lives and to talk to you about their experiences.

Reactions to an illness can happen at any time. Some children display behavior problems early in the illness while others show problems later. Sometimes children don't misbehave until their parents feel better and are past the worst phases of cancer diagnosis and treatment. With parental help, most children cope well throughout most of the illness, and most grow to be stronger people because of it.

If your plan doesn't work...

Review the points in the section *What You Can Do to Help* (pages 52–56). If you've tried everything and the children are still having trouble getting along in normal daily living, reread the section *When to Get Professional Help* (pages 50–51) and take steps to get some form of counseling.

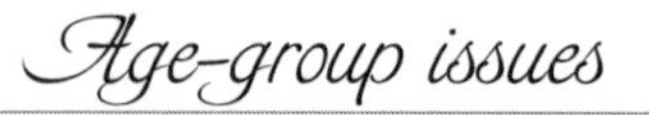

Children of different ages and developmental levels have different expectations and needs. Here is a list of thoughts and concerns common to three broad groupings: ages 2 to 5, 6 to 12, and adolescents.

Issues for toddlers and children (2 to 5)

- Fear of being separated from a parent or someone they love
- Fear of "catching" the disease
- May think they caused the illness by misbehaving
- May become angry because they receive less attention
- Confusion about the disease, its cause, treatments, and what it does to the person with cancer
- Magical thinking about the person with cancer getting better

WAYS TO HELP

Be honest, don't exceed the child's attention span, and repeat and reinforce security and love for the child. Try to limit the number of babysitters.

Issues for children of primary school age (6 to 12)

- Fear of changes in family, lifestyles, activities, and security
- Fear of embarrassment over being different from friends and possible guilt over being embarrassed
- May ask for details about the person with cancer's condition and treatment
- Fear of "catching" the disease

- Anger over limitations imposed on them by the illness
- May be confused about how to explain the illness to friends
- May question the role of religion

WAYS TO HELP

Be clear that cancer isn't contagious and the children or their behavior did not "cause" the person's cancer. Let children know in advance about "babysitters" who may come in to watch them. Try to maintain regular routines with different adults watching them. Keep the child's school informed about the situation. It may help to have the child come along to treatment or to talk with the doctors and nurses who are taking care of the person with cancer.

Issues for adolescents

- May resent and/or fear changes in family, lifestyles, and activities
- Any deception will cause distrust—tell the truth at all costs
- May feel guilty about wanting to exert independence at a time when they are needed to help at home
- May be embarrassed by being different from peers or by the physical appearance of the person with cancer
- Confusion may happen because, at a time when they want and expect more control over their lives, this illness reinforces their lack of control
- Issues of religion may surface

For this group, rapid and confusing change is already a part of their lives as they make the transition from being dependent children to being adults. The additional confusion that comes from a serious illness in the family only adds to their stress.

WAYS TO HELP

Adolescents sometimes feel more comfortable talking to someone outside of their families about their feelings—such as a friend, teacher, or counselor. Keep the school informed of the situation. Show your willingness to talk about religion. Encourage adolescents to maintain hobbies, sports, or other activities. Also, be careful not to load down an adolescent with too much responsibility—give him or her some breathing room.

Coordinating Care from One Treatment Setting to Another

Understanding the Situation

People with cancer are usually hospitalized more than once during different episodes of the illness, and they may also spend time in a rehabilitation center or nursing home. As you work out routines and schedules and learn to manage different symptoms and problems at home, you will want to see many of these same routines followed as closely as possible whenever the person stays somewhere else.

Telling the health care staff what works at home helps them deliver the best care in their setting. Requesting that certain routines be followed increases the chances of continuing your plans successfully. If you don't inform the health care staff, particularly the admitting physician, about these needs, then the person with cancer may end up with unmanaged symptoms.

For example, if you and the person with cancer have settled on a schedule of pain pills that keeps the pain away and also keeps him or her fully alert, you don't want to see this regimen abandoned when he or she is hospitalized. This can happen, especially if the person is put in a different hospital from the one where the doctor who originally prescribed the pain medicine works. Another example is when a different doctor prescribes additional doses of a pain medicine. The person with cancer might have been seen by medical oncologists for months but was seen later by a radiation oncologist and received a higher dose of pain medicine. If he or she returns to the medical oncologist, the new pain prescriptions need to be explained. Whoever admits the person to the hospital or any new setting needs to know exactly what drugs are given at home, when they are given, and how effective they are.

Maintaining medication schedules is not the only concern. Equipment that works well at home (such as a certain walker or toilet seat) should be used in the hospital or other setting. Personal care preferences and routines should also be known and followed, if possible.

Your goal is to:

- continue helpful procedures and routines as the person with cancer moves from one treatment setting to another

When to Get Professional Help

If the problems in coordinating care are making the person with cancer very uncomfortable, and you have tried the ideas in this chapter without success, then ask to speak to a nurse supervisor or physician. Explain the problems you are having and why you are concerned, and ask for their help. If you still have problems, ask to talk to the patient advocate at the hospital. Patient advocates are on the staff of most hospitals, and their job is to help when you feel the hospital is not doing its job.

What You Can Do to Help

First, review the kinds of personal help, special equipment, diet, and other needs of the person with cancer. Then plan how you will ensure these needs are met in the new treatment setting.

Take some time to prepare answers to the following questions:

- What kinds of personal help does the person with cancer need? Examples:
    - help in taking medicines
    - help with medical procedures (such as ostomy or catheter care)
    - help with eating
    - help getting out of bed
    - help with walking
    - help going to the toilet
    - help with sleeping
    - help with bathing
- Is any special equipment needed, such as a commode or special mattress?

- Is there a special diet to be followed and does the person have food likes or dislikes?
- What kinds of things make the day more enjoyable for him or her, such as listening to music, watching television, reading the newspaper, or getting the mail?
- What does he or she worry about, and how can the staff be most comforting and reassuring?
- What other facts would you want to tell to those who will be helping the person with cancer?

Plan how the needs of the person with cancer will be met in the new treatment setting

The person's needs can be grouped into two categories: *continuing medical care* and *continuing familiar routines.*

CONTINUING MEDICAL CARE IN NEW TREATMENT SETTINGS

Plan how you can continue the same schedule of medicines to prevent distressing symptoms or other discomforts.

Give a list to the admitting doctor or nurse of the names of and times of day that medicines are given (Table 1). This ensures that medicines are given close to the same times as usual. It is especially important to do this for medicines that were originally ordered as "prn" or "as needed," but you have learned that a certain timing or routine is most helpful. If you tell this routine to the admitting physician and nurse, they can write orders so that the routine is changed as little as possible.

List the food or liquid that is served with the pills alongside the medication schedule. The staff can then write in their plans "give with milk" or "serve with a small amount of applesauce."

Write down in what form the pill is given–for example, if it is crushed or mixed with applesauce. If pills are crushed, then they are crushed into something such as Maalox or applesauce. Or a suppository may be used. If you write these instructions down, there will be no confusion.

Ask the admitting physician to order a laxative or enema for the same day you would give one at home if no bowel movement has occurred. Unfortunately, it often takes a few days to notice constipation at a new setting. If the same elimination routine is followed at home, less discomfort will result.

Ask the nurses to write the bowel elimination routine in the nursing care plan. Many times the family gives key information to the nurse who admits the person with cancer to the hospital or new setting, but it is written down in a long admission note, which may not be read by the nursing staff when problems occur. However, if this information is written on the nursing care plan, it will be noticed and used in caring for the patient.

Ask the nurses to order a bedside commode or raised toilet seat if either is used at home. Upon admission, the staff does not know how difficult it is for the person with cancer to get to the commode. If you used a bedside commode or a raised toilet seat at home, then it is likely they will be needed in the hospital too. Tell the admitting physician or nurse about this so that the right equipment can be available when it is needed.

Ask the doctor to order a soft or blenderized diet if it is preferred. This ensures that meals are edible, especially if a sore mouth or mouth ulcers are a problem.

Table 1. Sample medication chart to give to admitting nurse or doctor

Medication	Dosage	Time of Day	Food or Liquid Served	Form
Amoxicillin	250 mg every 8 hours	12:00 A.M. 8:00 A.M. 4:00 P.M.	Small amount of applesauce	Tablet crushed into applesauce
Phenergan	25 mg every 4–6 hours	As needed	Before meals	Suppository
Tamoxifen	10 mg twice a day	10:00 A.M. 5:00 P.M.	Large glass of water	Tablets

Ask the doctor to write the mouth care regimen used at home in the admitting orders. If warm salt rinses or baking soda rinses are a routine at home, then ask that they be a part of the doctor's admitting orders. The staff will then give these items to the person and help with rinsing. Otherwise, it is up to you or the person with cancer to bring the salt or baking soda in and remember to rinse after meals and at bedtime.

CONTINUING FAMILIAR ROUTINES IN NEW TREATMENT SETTINGS

Bring the mail and newspaper. Familiar routines are not limited to medicines and personal care. Staying in touch with one's home can also bring a sense of comfort and control.

Bring musical tapes, relaxation tapes, or radios that are used at home. Distractions, no matter how short, are important for relief of anxiety or tension that goes along with being in the hospital or nursing center. Music or relaxation tapes can be brought in and played for enjoyment and distraction. Radios are not usually available in these settings, so you may have to bring one in for the person to listen to favorite news and music programs. Earphones can be used if he or she is in a semiprivate room.

Bring turbans, scarves, caps, or head coverings worn at home. Looking presentable can be very important to someone who is sick.

Bring in aids for walking such as canes or walkers.

Bring in aids for comfort and sleep such as small pillows or favorite blankets.

If a special mattress is needed, ask for it ahead of time. Many people like the contour of foam "egg shell" mattresses. Other mattresses are filled with air or water, especially if skin care is a problem. If a special mattress is used at home, ask that the same type be used in the new setting. If you ask ahead of time, it's more likely to be on the bed before admission. Even if it isn't, having asked beforehand may help in getting it sooner.

Possible Obstacles

Here are some things that others have said stood in their way of coordinating care:

"I expect the doctor to coordinate care."

The doctor may not know about what helped at home or at another treatment setting. You have to tell him or her.

Give the doctor a list of medicines, how they are taken (such as pills, suppositories, or injections, and so on), and times they are taken, and a list of what helps the person swallow medicine. (Refer to Table 1 on page 65.)

Doctors also don't know the specific bowel elimination plan, mouth care routines, diets, or equipment that helped the person with cancer at home. If you ask the doctor to write this information as medical orders, then the nurses will follow the orders.

"I don't want the staff to think I'm bossing them around."

Nurses and doctors will welcome your information. These facts are important to the person's comfort and health. **Having written lists helps the nurses and doctors when they write this information in the medical record and order diet, equipment, and medicines.**

"They don't have enough staff to do all the things I am asking for."

You have a right to expect good care. If your requests are important for the care and comfort of the person with cancer, you may have to "make a fuss." You may also have to visit often to be sure things are happening as they should. Care should never be compromised because of insufficient staffing.

Think of other obstacles that could interfere with carrying out your plan

What additional roadblocks could get in the way of doing the things recommended in this chapter? For example, will the person with cancer cooperate? How will you explain what is needed to other people? Do you have the time and energy to carry out the plan?

Develop plans for getting around these roadblocks using the six problem-solving steps discussed in the first section of this book (see pages xi–xvi).

Carrying Out and Adjusting Your Plan

Carrying out your plan

If possible, write your requests before the person you are caring for goes to a new treatment setting, and give them to the staff before or when he or she arrives. If the transfer happens too quickly for you to do this ahead of time, take your lists to the new medical staff as soon as possible after the transfer.

Checking on results

Check with the person you are caring for about whether the lists you made are being followed. Ask the nurses to see a copy of their orders, and check to be sure your lists are included.

If your plan doesn't work...

If you are having difficulty giving your information to the right person, or if the staff is not using your information, ask a member of the staff to help you. Involve them in solving the problem of coordinating care. Social workers are often good sources of help. They know the doctors and nurses and can give them your lists and ideas.

You can also ask to talk with the charge nurse or head nurses about your concerns. If you still are unhappy about how care is being coordinated, ask to speak with the head nurse or patient advocate. Usually, such steps are not needed because the health care staff will want to continue using methods that worked at home to manage symptoms.

MANAGING CARE

Getting Help from Community Agencies and Volunteer Groups

Understanding the Situation

Many people with cancer and their families do not fully understand the services that are available to help them in their own communities and in the hospitals and clinics where they receive treatment. As a result, they struggle alone with their problems when there are people and organizations able and willing to help. Finding out about these services and how to qualify for and use them is a challenge.

Even if you don't need to use these services right now, knowing they are available is like having "money in the bank." It can reassure you that there are resources available to help when you need them.

This chapter discusses the types of services people with cancer sometimes need and that are available in most communities: help with transportation and driving, home nursing visits, help with meals and household chores, and hospice care for advanced cancer. Understanding how to find and use these services will give you skills you can use to find additional community services.

We recommend you learn about available services before problems arise. You can do a more complete job of learning about these services when you are not under pressure to deal with a serious problem. If you need these services later, you will know what to do and where to go immediately.

Your goals are to:

- know who to ask about community services
- know what services are available in your community or hospital
- know how to qualify for and use those services

When to Get Professional Help

If you are having difficulty arranging for the help you need, ask to speak to a social worker. Social workers are professionals experienced in finding help from community agencies and volunteer groups.

Most hospitals, local offices of aging, health, and human services agencies have social workers on their staff. Ask a doctor or nurse at the hospital where the person with cancer is receiving treatment to arrange for you to talk to a social worker.

What You Can Do to Help

Getting help in finding community services

There are a number of places you can go for help in finding and using services in the community. We suggest you try all of these since one may list something that others do not.

Ask social workers. They are professionals with knowledge, skills, and experience in finding community services to help people with cancer and their families deal with illness-related problems. They deal regularly with community agencies and know not only what services are available, but also which agencies provide the best services. You are entitled to talk to hospital social workers when the person with cancer is a patient in the hospital or is coming for treatments at the hospital. Usually you can call the social workers directly without being referred, but in some hospitals they prefer that the doctor make a referral. To get a referral, tell the doctor or nurse that you want to talk to a social worker. If a knowledgeable social worker is not available, ask an oncology nurse to help you.

Ask knowledgeable people in your community. People in certain positions in a community know a lot about which local agencies and organizations provide services. Clergy are usually well informed on these matters, as well as local elected officials and officers of local community organizations such as the United Way. If these people can't help you directly, they usually know who to ask.

Ask about agencies that help you find services. Most communities have agencies that specialize in helping people find the services they need. They have different titles in different communities or parts of the country, but some examples are local offices of the American Cancer Society, United Way, Area Agencies for the Aging, religious agencies such as Catholic Charities or the local Councils of Churches, and community mental health centers. Hospital social workers know about these agencies in your area and can explain what they do.

Look in the GUIDE TO HUMAN SERVICES *section (or similar title) of local telephone books.* Most local telephone books contain sections listing community agencies and the services they provide. Often this is in a separate section and is printed on a different color paper to set it off from the rest. Often the pages are blue. Look at the table of contents in the beginning of your local telephone book for the Human Services section.

Transportation and driving

Getting transportation to and from treatments or medical appointments can be difficult. Look for help if any of the following conditions exist:

- You cannot drive the person to appointments.
- You cannot get the person from the house to the car, or they cannot sit for the length of the trip.
- You are falling asleep at the wheel, the trip is too long, you hesitate to drive, or you fear the trip.
- You cannot miss work or give up the money from work hours to take the time needed for the trip, the waiting, the appointment, and the return trip.

Possible solutions to transportation problems

Ask family or friends for help with driving. The more specific you are, the more likely that others will understand your request and be able to judge what is involved with their service. Tell them:

- what days of the week you could use drivers
- how long the trip takes each way
- whether he or she can be dropped off
- whether someone will meet him or her at the door
- how much parking costs are
- how long the usual appointment lasts
- whether he or she needs help getting in and out
- whether a wheelchair is involved
- whether money is available for their gasoline expenses

Ask a family member or a friend to arrange transportation. If you don't want to ask for help, have someone else ask for you. Having a scheduler is especially helpful when the person with cancer must go for treatments every day or every week. Church groups often arrange transportation for members and may be willing to arrange drivers for nonmembers.

Ask your local American Cancer Society (800-ACS-2345) if they have a volunteer transportation program. Many offices of the American Cancer Society run transportation programs. Volunteer drivers are trained to help the person with cancer, and their service is free. In addition, the schedule of drivers is arranged for you. If your local office does not have such a program, then ask if the next nearest office has a transportation program. Sometimes volunteer drivers who live close to your county are willing to help with driving.

Ask local service clubs, such as the Elks, Lions Club, Masons, or American Legion, if they or their auxiliaries could schedule drivers or help with transportation expenses. There are several organizations that have volunteers who drive people with serious illnesses to medical appointments. This varies from community to community.

Check with your local organizations. Ask the club or their auxiliaries to assign one member to schedule drivers. Some service groups raise money to help with medical expenses. If a relative or friend belongs to such a group in your community, ask him or her to explain your needs.

Ask a social worker, caseworker, or nurse to recommend paid drivers to you. Do not try to get paid help on your own. Ask the social worker or nurse involved in caring for the person for guidance in finding paid help. They understand the kind of help you need, and they have had experience with different agencies and ways to get help.

Ask if the treatment center or medical clinic has their own transportation van service. Some centers offer free transportation to and from chemotherapy or radiation appointments. Usually these are van services, and the person must be prepared to spend half the day at the treatment site. Many enjoy riding with others who are receiving similar treatments.

Use a county medical van. If treatments are within the same county, a county van service may help you. If treatments are outside of the county, ask if the transportation service crosses county lines.

Home nursing services

There are three types of nursing services: visits from registered nurses, visits from private duty nurses, and visits from nurses' aides.

Ask about visits from registered nurses. The doctor can prescribe home visits by registered nurses to do skilled nursing procedures and to give certain chemotherapy drugs at home. They can come to the home for short procedures, such as taking blood or urine samples to the laboratory for you or helping with dressing changes on a wound, ostomy opening, or IV site. Nurses can come out once a week or every day to do "skilled nursing procedures," such as teaching how to care for an IV line, how to change a dressing on a wound, or how to take medicines correctly. Their visits are often short (about an hour), and the cost is covered by insurance after they get approval from a doctor to visit. They can also arrange for others to visit, if needed, such as nurses' aides, social workers, speech therapists, occupational therapists, and physical therapists.

Some agencies send a nurse out just to do a blood draw or some other short task. The cost of this visit is seldom covered by insurance, but the fees are usually low. Ask the nurses or social workers to recommend an agency you can call about this service.

Chemotherapy nurses can come to the home when it is difficult to travel to the clinic. These nurses can be the same ones you see at the clinic or doctor's office where chemotherapy is given, or they can be employed by a visiting nurse agency. Ask the clinic nurses about this possibility.

Ask about visits from private-duty nurses. You can arrange for private-duty nurses without a doctor's approval. Visits from these nurses can last as long as you want. However, many agencies want a minimum visit of four hours. For example, some families find it helpful to arrange for eight hours of overnight care. The cost of this service is usually not covered by insurance, but be sure to ask in case it is.

Ask about visits from nurses' aides. You can sometimes arrange for nurses' aides for personal care services without a doctor's approval. However, it is best to check with a social worker to be sure the agency sending the aide is reliable. Nurses' aides can visit when you do not need help from a registered nurse. Nurses' aides, also called attendants, can help with bathing, walking, shopping, cooking, and light household chores.

Help with meals and household chores

Call your local Area Agency on the Aging, which will be listed in the phone book. Most cities and small towns have home-delivered meals. Many of these programs are for senior citizens. If you are under 65 years old, you may still be able to qualify, so call and ask. The cost of the service varies, and you may be eligible for reduced rates. Usually a hot lunch is delivered, along with a cold meal to be eaten later in the day. Special diets are available, such as diabetic, low-sodium, and low-fat diets. If these services are not listed under "Meals" in the phone book, look for the Area Agency on the Aging, which often provides these services or knows who does.

Ask about agencies that help with meal preparation. Some agencies have programs where a worker or nurses' aide comes to the home a few times a week to shop for food and supplies, run errands, prepare meals, and do light housekeeping.

Ask church groups or neighbors to organize a small home helper group. Many churches are happy to do this and can do yard work, window washing, or other chores. Sometimes they arrange for the youth group to get involved.

Hospice care

Hospice care is available when the person with cancer does not want any more treatment to extend life and wants the disease to take its natural course. It is also available for when physicians decide that treatments are not successful, they have nothing new to offer, and therefore recommend that treatments be stopped. When this happens, hospice is available to help the person with cancer have a comfortable, natural death.

Hospice programs help people whose life expectancy has been certified by a doctor to be six months or less. Their services are available in all cities and most small towns and rural areas. Hospices are often run by the local home health or visiting nurse agencies. Services are usually paid by insurance and Medicare.

In hospice programs, a team of professionals visit the home to help the family keep the person comfortable and to give physical care such as administering pain medicine, bathing, and help with toileting. Hospice workers are skilled in controlling pain and in managing symptoms caused by advanced cancer. They can also give emotional and spiritual support to the person with cancer and family, if wanted. Volunteers may help by coming to the home to give the family a chance to rest.

In most hospice programs, people with cancer receive care at home, though they may go to a hospital or residential care facility for short periods when special care is needed or to give the family relief from caregiving. In a few hospices people with cancer are not at home. They live in a special building and receive all care from special hospice staff.

Finding hospice care

Ask a cancer doctor, nurse, or social worker to give you a list of local hospices. Hospice services are also listed in the yellow pages of the telephone book. Agencies that will know about hospices in your community are the American Cancer Society, the Area Office on Aging, the local Visiting Nurse Association, your state's home care association, and the National Hospice and Palliative Care Association. See the *Resource Guide* at the end of this book for national contact information. State and local agencies are listed in the white and blue pages of your telephone book.

Possible Obstacles

Here are some things that others have said stood in their way of using community services:

"I don't want to ask for help. If people want to help, they'll offer."

Some people feel their friends and relatives should volunteer to help without being asked. If you feel this way, think back to people you knew who were sick and how difficult it sometimes was to find the time or inclination to volunteer to help. The fact that people don't volunteer doesn't mean that they would not help. Family and friends will probably welcome the opportunity to help if asked because they know that they are meeting a specific need. The chapter *Understanding Caregiving* (pages 32–45) has ideas to make helping enjoyable for everyone.

"No one around here can help drive. They don't have the time or the money for gas. Some don't even have cars or they work or are too busy with their families."

You don't know who can drive until you ask. Ask other people to help you find drivers. Also, retirees and those who are temporarily unemployed might have the time to give to help you solve this problem.

Carrying Out and Adjusting Your Plan

Carrying out your plan

Don't wait! Start learning now before you need information about how community agencies and volunteer groups can help you. This will be valuable information that you can use when you need it.

If you have trouble getting the information you need, ask someone to help you. Talk to a social worker at the hospital, the Area Office on Aging, or in community social service and health agencies. They have had a great deal of experience with these problems and can often be creative in helping you to get the help you need.

If your plan doesn't work...

If you are having some success but not as much as you would like, you may be expecting too much progress too soon. Be patient and keep trying. It often takes time to learn how to use community agencies and volunteer groups.

If you are feeling worn down by your problems, ask someone else to help you work out a solution. Sometimes people who are not directly involved can see new ways to deal with the problem.

Social workers have the most experience with these problems. If the social worker to whom you talked was not helpful, ask to talk to another social worker.

MANAGING CARE

Getting Information from Medical Staff

Understanding the Situation

Over the course of the illness, you will need a great deal of information to do your job as family caregiver. Some of this information is complicated, and often it must come from different sources. Therefore, it is not surprising that many family caregivers have difficulty getting the information they need. This chapter helps you deal with this problem by showing you an orderly sequence of steps to go through in getting medical information.

Two things to keep in mind about requesting medical information:

1. It is usually reasonable to assume the medical staff wants to help you and would like to give you the information you need.

2. Often certain staff members can't answer your questions because each medical care organization has its own rules about who knows what and who is allowed to give information to people with cancer and caregivers. One doctor's office has different rules from another doctor's office. One hospital differs from another, and even within the same hospital there are often different rules for inpatient (patients who stay overnight) and outpatient (patients who come and go in the same day) departments, different rules in surgery and in oncology, and so on. What this means is that you have to learn who knows what and who can tell you what for each new office, service, or hospital you deal with.

What information can you ask for?

Family caregivers should have all the information they need to provide the best possible care at home. There are five kinds of information that you need:

1. an understanding of the condition—What is it? What causes it? Who is most likely to have it? What can family caregivers expect to accomplish in dealing with the condition?
2. when to call for professional help
3. what you can do to deal with and prevent the condition
4. obstacles that might interfere
5. how to carry out and monitor your plan

You need all of this information if you are to meet your caregiving responsibilities. Feel free to ask for information and to persist until you have it.

Your goal is to get the medical information you need as quickly and efficiently as possible and with as little stress as possible for both yourself and the medical staff.

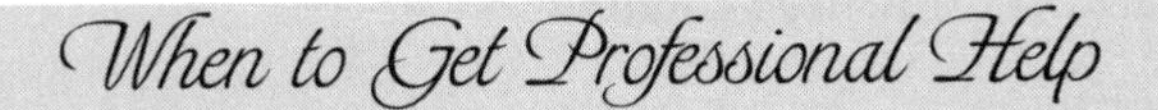

Whom to call for help

If you feel the situation is an emergency and you cannot get the information you need, then call the doctor or an emergency room. Be sure the person you talk to understands that you feel this is an emergency. To do this, use the word "emergency" in your question, and then be persistent until you have the information you need.

Here are some examples of phrasing you might use:

"I have an emergency and need to talk to a doctor." (Be prepared to answer the question *"What is the emergency?"*)

"I have a question about ____________________ and I'm not sure if this is really an emergency or not. Who can help me?"

"I'm very concerned about ________________________. I think it may be an emergency. Can you help me?"

What You Can Do to Help

There are three things you can do to improve your ability to get information you need. The following order is recommended.

1. Be sure your questions are phrased clearly.
2. Learn who can answer your questions.
3. Ask the questions yourself or have the person with cancer get the information you need.

1. Be sure your questions are phrased clearly.

Know exactly what information you need, and state your questions clearly.

Ask yourself "What do I need to know to do my job as a home caregiver?" This question is one of the best ways to begin deciding what other questions to ask to give you the information that you need. This focuses your attention on what is most important. Otherwise, you may find yourself asking a lot of questions without finding out what you really need to know.

When you ask questions, first say what you need to know and why you need to know it. It is much easier for someone else to understand your question if you start with a clear statement of the information you need. Then your listener will be able to understand the rest of what you say. For example, let's assume that the person you are caring for had malaria when he was in the service. You noticed that some of the symptoms after chemotherapy were similar to malaria, and this made you worried that the malaria was returning. When you ask your question, start by asking if any of his symptoms could be due to malaria. Say that the reason you are concerned is that he had malaria when he was in the service, and the symptoms after chemotherapy are very similar. The listener then knows both what you want to know and why.

Write out your questions and check them with other people. Keep a list of questions you want to ask at the next doctor visit or home health nurse visit. Writing down your questions beforehand is one of the best ways to be sure you are being clear. Having a nurse or social worker read your list before you see your doctor is a good way to check on your clarity. If you get flustered, which happens to many people, then you can read your questions.

2. Learn who can answer your questions.

Different people can give you different kinds of information, and this can vary with different doctors, hospitals, and clinics. You need to know who can tell you what for each new treatment setting.

Learn which staff members give different kinds of information to people with cancer. The best way to find this out is to ask a medical staff person such as a nurse, social worker, or physician. Secretarial staff are less likely to know this, but sometimes they can be helpful. Nurses or social workers are usually a good resource.

A good way to ask is to start your question with "Who can tell me ... ?" For example, "Who can tell me when my husband will be discharged" or "Who can tell me when my mother's treatments are scheduled?"

Be prepared to learn the rules about who can give you what information for every new group of health staff that you deal with. It is a good idea to ask these questions early, when you begin working with a new treatment team. That way you can avoid information problems later.

Be persistent! Pleasant persistence almost always pays off. If medical staff say they don't know or can't tell you, then ask who can. You may have to ask several people, but don't feel you are getting the run-around. Medical care is often complicated, which means that getting information about it can be complicated, too. Don't get discouraged. You have a right to all of the information you need to be the best possible caregiver. Getting information becomes easier and easier the better you understand the medical care system.

(See page 85 for a list of the types of information that different medical professionals can usually give you.)

3. Ask the questions yourself or have the person with cancer get the information you need.

Ask the questions yourself. Have a clear idea of what you need to know. Ask or read your questions. Ask follow-up questions until you are very clear about the answer you received.

Ask a nurse, social worker, or other member of the health care team to get the information you need. You may need to ask someone else to get information for you because you don't have the time to find the right person. It could be because the medical person you need to talk to is not available when you need the information, or it could be that he or she gives you an answer, but the answer doesn't contain the information you need. If any of these things happen, a good strategy is to ask a nurse or social worker to ask your questions for you. Nurses and social workers understand medical terminology and how medical organizations work. They are also usually good at explaining these things to nonmedical people. Choose nurses or social workers with whom you feel comfortable, and tell them what information you need and why you can't get it yourself. Then ask for their help.

Ask the person with cancer to get the information you need. The person with cancer sees all the people on the health care team and can be helpful in getting information that you need as a caregiver. However, people with cancer may have other things on their minds or be tired when they see the members of their health care team, so you may want to write down your questions, and you may also want to ask one of the staff (such as a nurse or social worker) to remind the person with cancer to ask the questions.

Sometimes the person with cancer doesn't want to ask questions because the answers may be upsetting. In this case, you may want to ask questions when you are alone with the doctor or nurse.

Possible Obstacles

What could prevent you from carrying out your plan to improve your ability to get information you need?

"My questions are stupid."

No questions are stupid. You and the medical staff want to give the best possible care to the person with cancer. To do this, you need to know what to do and why. Therefore, it is the medical staff's job to answer your questions and to educate you.

"I feel confused by the health care system."

Medical staff use unfamiliar words, have peculiar titles, and are organized into groups with unfamiliar names. It is not surprising that many people with cancer and their families are confused. It can be almost as confusing as going to a foreign country. What many people do when they go to a foreign country is to get a guide who speaks their language and the language of the new country. This is a good model for learning about the health care system. Your guides can be health care staff who know the system—nurses and social workers are often good guides. Ask them to explain the system to you: what the titles mean, what the different groups do, and what medical terms mean. As you learn about the system, you will soon be using the medical terms yourself and finding your way around like a veteran.

"I feel intimidated by medical staff."

Some people feel that medical staff are so important or so busy that they should not take up their valuable time with questions. This is not so! Medical staff are there to help people with cancer. To do this, the staff must give family caregivers the information they need to care for the person with cancer at home.

"If I need to know something, the doctor will tell me."

Although the doctor will try to tell you everything you need to know, he or she can't always remember what you were told before, may assume that someone else told you, or may simply forget to tell you certain things. So you need to tell the doctor what your needs are.

"If I ask too many questions, the staff will think I'm a nuisance, and then they won't take good care of the person I am helping."

It is unlikely that the staff will think you are a nuisance. However, even if they do, this would not affect how they treat the person with cancer. Medical professionals are trained to treat everyone to the best of their ability no matter what they think about the person. To do otherwise would be malpractice.

Think of other obstacles that could interfere with carrying out your plan

What additional roadblocks could get in the way of doing the things recommended in this chapter? For example, will the person with cancer cooperate? Will other people help? How will you explain your needs to medical staff? Do you have the time and energy to carry out the plan?

Develop plans for getting around these roadblocks using the six problem-solving steps outlined at the beginning of this book (see pages xi–xvi).

Carrying Out and Adjusting Your Plan

Carrying out your plan

Ask questions. The more questions you ask, the easier it becomes. In the beginning you may want to read your questions. Also practice beforehand what you will say. Set deadlines for getting certain information.

Checking on results

Keep track of the number of times you have problems getting information you need. Don't expect perfect results right away. However, over time you will improve your ability to get the information you need.

If your plan doesn't work...

If you are having some success, but not as much as you would like, you may be expecting too much progress too soon. Be patient and keep trying. The medical care system is complicated, and it takes time to master it.

If you feel medical staff are not giving you the information you need, your next step can be to make an appointment with the physician who has responsibility for the person's care and ask him or her your questions. Explain the problems you have had in getting information and ask how to avoid these problems in the future. (Note that you may be charged for this appointment, and many insurers will not pay for appointments with care persons. It is best to ask about this when making the appointment. If you cannot afford to pay, you can ask to have the fee waived or you can ask if your meeting can be scheduled as part of the person's regular meeting with the physician.) Don't be angry and don't be intimidated. Being angry only makes the other person angry too, and being intimidated means that you won't explain the situation clearly. A calm, objective approach works best.

Most hospitals have patient advocates or similar staff members. These people are familiar with problems in the hospital as well as with how to deal with those problems. They can help you to get information and in addition, they can help to change the way the hospital operates. You may help future patients by telling patient advocates about problems you are having.

As a last resort, the person with cancer always has the right to change doctors or treatment settings. If he or she is considering that, be sure the new setting will give the support you need.

Kinds of information that different medical professions can usually give you

Physicians: treatment plans, prognosis (the likelihood of cure or remission and the usual course of the disease), how often the person will be evaluated, how often he or she needs to see a doctor, when he or she should be admitted to a hospital, what medicines should be taken and when, results of tests, and whether the medicine is working

Nurses: management of side effects of treatments, appointment schedules, nutrition information, results of some tests (this depends on the doctor or hospital policies), and how and when to take medications

Social workers: help in dealing with family and emotional problems, how to arrange for medical care at home, how to be admitted to a nursing home or hospice program, how to get financial help or whether the person with cancer qualifies for different government programs

This list is a good starting point for getting information, but be prepared for lots of exceptions. Hospital physicians have different titles such as "attending," "fellow," "resident," and "consultant" as well as different types of specialties such as "surgeon," "oncologist," "radiation therapist," "pathologist," and so on. Depending on your medical needs, physicians with different titles and specialties have different responsibilities and can give you different kinds of information. When several physicians are involved, one member of the team will be coordinating the care. In this case, ask who is the coordinating physician.

Emotional Conditions

This section helps you deal with emotional conditions such as anxiety and depression, not only in the person with cancer but in yourself as well.

The information in this section fits most situations, but yours may be different. If the doctor or nurse tells you to do something else, follow what they say. If you think there may be a medical emergency, see the When to Get Professional Help section of each chapter.

This section explains situations faced by many caregivers and people with cancer. Encourage the person with cancer to read this information, and then you can work together as a team.

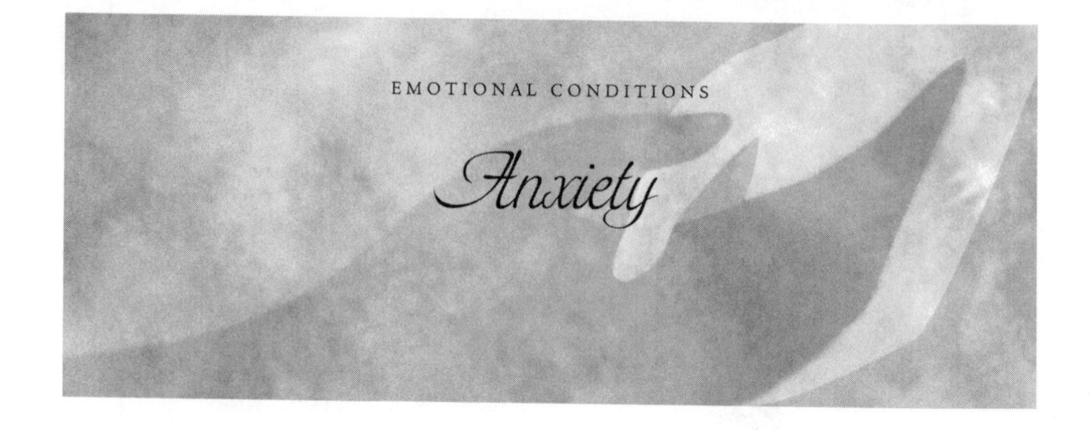

Understanding the Condition

During a stressful illness such as cancer, the person with cancer often becomes anxious, as do his or her family and friends. Medical procedures or fear of the future may cause anxiety. Caregivers may worry about the person's illness and their own ability to cope effectively with caregiving. Sometimes the person with cancer's anxiety makes caregivers anxious. Poor communication between the person with cancer and family and friends can also be a source of anxiety for everyone. Therefore, read this chapter to help the person with cancer and also to help yourself.

What is anxiety?

Anxiety is a common and normal response to new or stressful situations. Everyone has felt worried at various times in their lives. For example, people often feel anxious or nervous before they interview for a new job, before talking to a group of people, or when they are worried about someone they love. Here are some different ways that people experience anxiety:

- nervousness
- tension
- panicky feelings
- confusion
- fear
- feeling something bad is going to happen
- feeling like "I'm losing control"
- anger or irritation

When you are anxious you may also have physical symptoms, such as:

- sweaty palms
- upset stomach
- tight feelings in your stomach
- shaking or tremors
- difficulty breathing
- racing pulse
- hot and flushed face
- diarrhea or constipation
- frequent urination
- headaches

Sometimes these feelings come and go fairly quickly. Other times these feelings last a long time.

Tension can sometimes help people. For example, many actors say that they have "butterflies in their stomach," or anxious moments, before they perform. Sometimes people actually enjoy the feelings of anxiety, like when they are watching a horse race or riding a roller coaster.

However, when these feelings are very strong and contain fearful thoughts, they interfere with everyday living. When they last a long time—such as more than a week—they can prevent people from doing things that are important to them. This is when people need to learn to manage their anxiety.

Recognizing when a person is anxious

One of the difficult things about anxiety is that people may not know when they're experiencing it. They may think that they are just worried. Before they realize what is happening, they are experiencing serious anxiety symptoms.

Sometimes people with cancer don't realize how anxious they are becoming, but family and friends do. Family and friends can help by pointing out what is happening early, and they can help the person with cancer control the anxiety before it gets out of hand.

Anxiety related to cancer

When people are told they have cancer, it often makes them feel anxious. Some feel afraid, nervous, and even overwhelmed. Others may feel panicky, as if they have lost control of their lives. These are normal reactions that may last from a few days to a few weeks.

Many people with cancer experience anxiety during their treatments. Anxiety can be caused by:

- fear of being a burden to family and friends
- fear of getting sicker and having a shorter life
- pain and discomfort
- a side effect of cancer treatment medicines
- worries about medical procedures

Anxiety can make physical symptoms more intense. For example, a person who is in pain usually reports more severe pain when he or she is feeling anxious. Although some anxiety is normal for people with cancer, it can become so severe that it interferes with their ability to cope with the illness. Anxiety may make some people reluctant to visit the doctor and may even make them think of dropping out of treatment. Severe anxiety can also seriously reduce the quality of life of people with cancer.

Controlling anxiety is primarily in the hands of the person with cancer. You can give encouragement and help.

Try not to feel guilty if, in spite of your best efforts, the person with cancer is very anxious. If the anxiety is severe, a professional may be needed who can use special techniques such as anti-anxiety medicines or stress management techniques.

What you can hope to accomplish

Since anxiety is a normal response to new or stressful situations, don't expect to totally eliminate all anxiety. What you and the person with cancer can do together is prevent anxiety from becoming so severe and so long lasting that it seriously degrades his or her quality of life or interferes with receiving needed cancer treatments.

Your goals are to:

- accept that some anxiety is both normal and understandable
- help the person with cancer get professional help for anxiety when necessary

- help the person with cancer learn about his or her anxiety and how to manage it as much as possible
- use the ideas in this chapter for yourself if anxiety is interfering with your ability to help your loved one

When to Get Professional Help

Urge the person with cancer to call the doctor, nurse, psychologist, or social worker for anxiety (or do so yourself) if he or she...

- ▲ **Is seriously considering dropping out of treatment.** Sometimes people skip treatments or avoid visits to the doctor because of anxiety.
- ▲ **Has a history of severe anxiety requiring professional help or therapy.** It is important for the health care team to know about any problems with anxiety in the past.
- ▲ **Has a much lower quality of life due to anxiety.** Professional help is needed if anxiety symptoms are interfering with daily activities or are very upsetting to the person with cancer.
- ▲ **Is becoming increasingly anxious.** Some people are hesitant to ask for help with emotional problems because they don't want to appear "crazy." They need to understand that being upset during a major illness is normal, as is seeking help for these problems.

Call the doctor, nurse, or social worker if any of the following symptoms persist for several days:

- ▲ **Severe problems with sleeping several days in a row.**
- ▲ **Feelings of dread and serious apprehension for several days.**
- ▲ **Trembling, twitching, and feeling "shaky."**
- ▲ **Fluttering stomach with nausea and diarrhea.**
- ▲ **Increased heart rate or feeling a rapid pulse.**
- ▲ **Wide mood swings that cannot be controlled.**
- ▲ **Shortness of breath.**

Some of these symptoms could be caused by cancer or side effects of the treatments as well as by anxiety. The physician treating the person with cancer can evaluate what is causing these symptoms.

It is best to start with the physician treating the cancer or a family physician who knows the person with cancer and the treatments he or she is receiving. Ask for an evaluation of possible causes of the anxiety and recommendations for treatment or referral.

Physicians can evaluate whether a change in the cancer treatment or medicines is needed or whether to prescribe antianxiety medicines. Physicians can also make referrals to mental health professionals such as psychologists, psychiatrists, social workers, and nurse counselors. If you are not sure whether professional help is needed, ask a nurse or social worker for guidance.

Also, be alert to whether family members need help because of anxiety. If their anxiety is severe, they may need help just as the person with cancer does.

What You Can Do to Help

If it's not an emergency, here are some things you can do working as a team with the person with cancer:

- find out what thoughts may be causing the anxiety
- encourage talking to someone who has been through the situation causing the anxiety
- engage in some pleasant, distracting activities
- add companionship
- encourage use of relaxation techniques
- ask a physician for an evaluation

Try to find out exactly what thoughts are making the person with cancer anxious. Understanding the thoughts that are causing the anxiety is the key to controlling it.

Anxiety has two parts: thoughts and feelings. Worried thoughts lead to nervous feelings. Nervous feelings can lead to more worried thoughts and so on. To stop this cycle, you first need to find out what thoughts are causing the anxiety and why those thoughts are making him or her nervous. For example, he or she may say going into the hospital is upsetting, but when you ask what it is about the hospital that makes it upsetting, you may learn that he or she is afraid of being left alone. On the other hand, another person may be concerned about paying the hospital bills. Sometimes you won't be able to find an exact reason; this is when professional help may be useful.

If the person is anxious about medical procedures, try to find out exactly what it is about the procedure that is upsetting. Is it needles, pain, being alone, being naked, being in an enclosed space? If the person cannot explain it, ask: "How would you change the procedures so they don't make you so upset?"

If the person is anxious about receiving medical information, try to find out exactly what kind of news would likely cause the person to be upset. Is it being told to have more treatments? Having to go into the hospital? The prospect of being unable to do certain things in the future?

It is important to be tactful and sensitive when asking these types of questions. Just talking about the upsetting event may make the person even more upset. Pay close attention to what the person is saying and allow him or her to finish without interruption. It may then be helpful to summarize what was said to show you understand. Being a good listener by itself can be helpful to the person with cancer by showing there is someone who understands his or her feelings. It also allows the anxious person to hear him or herself talk about the problem, which can help to put it in perspective.

Get the exact facts. Getting the facts can help a person feel less anxious. For example, if he or she is worried about whether the doctor will say that the disease has progressed, you may learn the doctor will not know whether the cancer is responding to treatment for another eight weeks. Or, if he or she is upset by needles, you may learn the test the doctor has ordered does not use needles.

Look for ways around the problem. When you get the facts, you may also discover there are ways to "get around" a problem that is making the person anxious. For example, if the anxiety is about needle sticks in the veins, blood could be drawn with a small prick on the finger. Or, if he or she is worried about being alone during chemotherapy or a test, you can plan to be with the person during that time.

Encourage the person with cancer to talk to someone who has been through a similar situation. It is often reassuring to hear about what happened to someone else and how that person reacted during a stressful experience. It helps the person with cancer to know he or she is not alone and that someone else got through it. This can make the future seem more manageable, even if the experience was difficult for the other person.

Carefully choose the person you talk to since some people can be more reassuring than others. In general, though, most people find talking to someone who has been through the same experience reduces worry and anxiety.

Most people who have made it through scary experiences are happy to talk to others about their experiences. The treatment team may be able to refer you to a person or to a support group where you can find a person who has had similar experiences.

Engage in some pleasant, distracting activities. Helping the person with cancer think about and do things that are pleasant and relaxing can help reduce anxiety.

There are many types of enjoyable activities that can be helpful to a person who is anxious, such as activities with other people, activities that give a sense of accomplishment, and activities that are especially involving that distract thoughts away from the anxiety-causing situation.

Increase companionship and time spent with friends and family who care. Being with family and friends who the person with cancer knows and enjoys is an excellent way to take attention away from what is causing the anxiety. It can also give family and friends the opportunity to express caring and love. Knowing other people care and are available to help when needed gives people strength and confidence in facing frightening experiences.

Encourage the person with cancer to use relaxation techniques. Relaxation is a skill that can be used to counteract anxiety. You can't be anxious and relaxed at the same time. When you do things that make the person with cancer feel relaxed, anxiety decreases.

There are many ways to feel more relaxed. Prayer or meditation helps many people when they are in tense situations. Many people are relaxed by certain kinds of music. Walking or mild exercise can also reduce anxiety and deep breathing repeatedly helps some people to relax their minds and bodies.

There are also special relaxation exercises and tapes that are available commercially. These programs teach relaxation as a skill. With practice, people can learn to relax their muscles more than they usually would. They can then learn to use this skill when they are in tense situations. Oncology nurses, doctors, psychologists, and social workers are often familiar with relaxation techniques and may be able to recommend a program, book, or audiocassette tape.

The last section of this chapter (pages 98–99) explains how to use and practice relaxation techniques. It is important people practice these skills because the better the person with cancer is at becoming relaxed, the better he or she will be able to control anxiety.

Ask a physician about anxiety and how to treat it. If anxiety does not improve in spite of your efforts to help, then you can encourage the person with cancer to discuss the problem with a physician. Contact the physician treating the cancer or a family physician who knows about the medical situation and treatments.

Physicians can help in three ways

1. They can assess whether side effects of the disease or treatments may be causing the anxiety. They can then consider changes in the treatment, if appropriate.
2. They can assess whether antianxiety medicines need to be prescribed. Antianxiety medicine should only be taken after consulting with a physician who is familiar with the cancer diagnosis and treatments. These medicines may cause problems when combined with other medicines.
3. They can assess whether referral to a mental health professional is needed. If so, they can help with a referral.

Possible Obstacles

Here are some obstacles that other people have faced in helping a person with cancer deal with anxiety:

"My problems are real. I have to face them even if they make me anxious."

Agree that the problems are real. A certain amount of anxiety about them is normal and understandable. However, research and experience shows severe anxiety interferes with the ability to solve problems. Managing anxiety makes problem solving easier.

"I can't stop the thoughts that make me anxious. They keep coming back and racing around my head."

It's scary to feel like you can't control your thoughts. However, there are some techniques to try which may reduce or even stop them. In the chapter on depression, there is a section on stopping negative thoughts (pages 107–111). These can also work for anxiety.

"Because I'm the caregiver, I feel like I have to help everyone else with their problems. I'm always tired and I'm becoming frustrated.".

Spending a lot of time with someone who is very anxious can be stressful and can also make you anxious. You need to take time for yourself—to deal with your own problems. Use ideas in this chapter and *Depression* (pages 100–113) for yourself, as well as for the person you are caring for. Try to involve as many people as possible in carrying out this plan. More support will help both of you.

Think of other obstacles that could interfere with carrying out your plan

What additional roadblocks could get in the way of doing the things recommended in this chapter? For example, will the person with cancer cooperate? Will other people help? How will you explain your needs to other people? Do you have the time and energy to carry out the plan?

Develop plans for getting around these roadblocks using the six problem-solving steps discussed in the first section of this book (see pages xi–xvi).

Carrying Out and Adjusting Your Plan

Carrying out your plan

Your first step is to talk this plan over with the person with cancer. You are a team. You need to agree on what you will do together to try to manage anxiety.

If you think anxiety is likely at certain times, make plans for what to do at these times to prevent anxiety from building up. It is always easier to help someone manage anxiety before it is serious and before he or she feels overwhelmed by it.

Stay alert to the possibility that professional help may be needed. Review regularly the questions in the *When to Get Professional Help* section of this chapter (pages 91–92). Seek help if the anxiety seriously interferes with the ability of the person with cancer to complete treatment or if it is seriously hurting his or her quality of life.

Checking on results

Talk regularly with the person with cancer about emotional feelings just as you do about physical symptoms. Some people find it helpful to rate their anxiety on a 10-point scale, with zero (0) being "no anxiety" and ten (10) being "the worst anxiety ever experienced." Keeping a daily log of anxiety levels takes a little extra effort, but by keeping track of it, you can deal with it before it gets serious, which can save a lot of energy later.

If your plan doesn't work...

Ask yourself if you are expecting change too fast. It usually takes time to change someone's anxiety level. Look for small improvements at first. Remember: Your efforts may be successful even if they just stop the anxiety from getting worse.

If these techniques do not seem to be helping and the person with cancer has been feeling anxious for several weeks, then you need to get professional help.

A relaxation technique

Many persons with cancer have found relaxation techniques helpful. These techniques can be used anytime—even for short periods of time. Try this exercise yourself to see how it feels and works for you. This will help you to support the person with cancer in using these techniques.

Practice relaxation once a day, but not within an hour after a meal since digestion may interfere with the ability to relax certain muscles. Practice this exercise when you are not feeling rushed. It may be helpful for you to read these instructions out loud to the person with cancer.

1. Sit quietly in a comfortable position (such as in an easy chair or sofa).
2. Close your eyes.
3. Deeply relax your muscles, beginning with the face and going throughout the entire body (neck, shoulders, chest, arms, hands, stomach, legs) and ending with the feet. Allow the tension to "flow out through your feet."

   Now concentrate your attention on your head, and relax your head even further by thinking, "I'm going to let all the tension flow out of my head. I'm letting go of the tension, and I'm letting warm feelings of relaxation smooth out the muscles in my head and face. I'm becoming more relaxed."

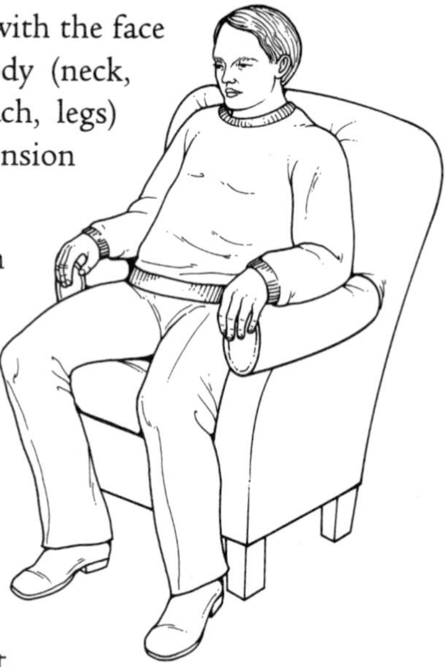

   Repeat these same steps for different parts of your body: your neck, shoulders, arms, hands, chest, abdomen, legs, and feet. Do this slowly—spend enough time to feel more relaxed before going on to the next part of the body.
4. When your body feels very relaxed, concentrate on your breathing. Become aware of how rhythmic and deep your breathing has become. Breathe slowly and deeply. Breathe through your nose.

As you breathe out, say the word "calm" silently to yourself. Slowly take a breath in. Now slowly let it out and silently say "calm" to yourself. Repeat this with every breath. It helps you to relax more if you concentrate on just this one word, "calm." Continue breathing deeply, becoming more and more relaxed.

5. Continue this exercise for 10 to 15 minutes. Remain relaxed and breathing slowly. At the end of the exercise, open your eyes slowly to become adjusted to the light in the room, and sit quietly for a few minutes.

When it is over, ask yourself how relaxed you became and if there were any problems. One problem can be drifting and distracting thoughts. If this happens at the next session, think to yourself, "Let relaxation happen at its own pace." If a distracting thought occurs, let it pass. Let it fly away like a bird. Don't fight it. Concentrate more on the word "calm." Let the thought drift by and repeat "calm" over and over again as your breathing gets slower and deeper—as you relax more and more.

Do these exercises regularly—once a day is best. In the beginning, it may help to have someone else give you the instructions. You can record these instructions on a tape recorder and play them when you are relaxing. If you prefer, you can record yourself giving the instructions and use that.

When practicing, choose a time when you will not be disturbed. Tell the other people in your household what you are doing and ask them to be quiet during the exercise.

After you become skilled at this exercise, you will find it is easy to apply when you are getting tense. For example, if you are feeling tense while waiting to see the doctor or for a treatment, you can easily close your eyes for a few minutes and use this exercise to relax and feel calm.

It's a good idea to learn this relaxation technique early—before anxiety becomes severe. It can then help to keep severe anxiety from happening.

Depression

Understanding the Condition

Many people with cancer become depressed at some time during their illness and family caregivers may become depressed as well. Caregivers often report depression was the most difficult symptom they had to deal with during the illness. It is during the early stages of depression you can be most helpful in controlling depression symptoms. If depression becomes severe, professional help will be needed, and you can help by encouraging the depressed person to get help. In all cases, working together as a team is essential. Paying attention to your own emotional needs is also important and allows you to give the best possible care.

The stress of dealing with an illness like cancer can cause many people to feel sad or "blue." Sometimes they are able to get over "the blues" after a short time. However, these feelings sometimes last a long time and can severely hurt their quality of life. When a person is sad, discouraged, pessimistic, or despairing for several weeks or months, and when these feelings interfere with being able to manage day-to-day affairs, we say he or she is suffering from depression. It can last a long time if the person doesn't do something to stop it. Depression can be significantly reduced by emotional support, counseling, and antidepression medicines.

In addition to feelings of sadness, symptoms sometimes include problems with appetite, sleeping, having the energy to do things, and concentrating or paying attention to things. Alcohol abuse, especially if it is new or worse since the illness, may be a sign of depression. Sometimes a depressed person also thinks about suicide as a way out.

If the person with cancer is depressed, he or she will have problems coping with their illness and the impact it has on their life.

Depression works like a downward spiral. The person feels down, so he or she doesn't put energy into solving problems. When the problems get worse, they can cause the person to feel worse. And so on and so on. Somehow this has to be interrupted. Some kind of change has to happen, or the person will have these feelings for a long time.

Depression can be a side effect of some medicines; it can be caused by unrelieved pain, or it can be caused by chemical imbalances in the body due to the cancer. When these happen, changes in medical treatments may help the depression.

In this chapter, we discuss some ways to tell when a depressed person must seek medical help. We also discuss some ways you can help a depressed person limit or manage depression. Your help is valuable to a person feeling depressed, but it is also important he or she practice certain self-help strategies. We discuss ways you and the person with cancer can work together as a team to deal with depression.

Some depression is a normal response to the stresses and uncertainties of chronic illness. Don't expect to get rid of all of these feelings. However, you can help limit the length and severity of depression.

As a caregiver, you can help prevent feelings of sadness or discouragement from becoming severe or continuing for long periods of time. Working as a team will help both of you keep depressed feelings under control. If the symptoms become severe, you can help the person with cancer get professional help.

Living with a person who is depressed can be stressful and can even lead to your becoming depressed. It is important to pay attention to your own emotional health if you are to do your best as a caregiver. You can also use the ideas in this chapter to help control your own depression.

Your goals are to:

- know when to get professional help
- take care of your own emotional needs when living with or caring for a person who is depressed
- work as a team with the person with cancer to manage depressed feelings and thoughts
- prevent or reduce depression

When to Get Professional Help

If any of the following is occurring, get assistance from a health professional:

- **The person with cancer is talking about hurting or killing himself or herself.** Suicide is not common among persons with cancer—but it is more common among depressed people. Therefore, anyone who talks about suicide should be taken seriously. If you are not sure, ask if he or she is thinking about suicide. Your asking won't make it more likely. If you think there is a possibility of suicide, this is a problem that requires professional assessment and help. Although it may be uncomfortable for you, seek professional assistance immediately.

- **He or she has experienced depression before this illness** and has had at least two of the following symptoms consistently during the past two weeks:

  - feeling sad most of the day
  - loss of interest in almost all daily activities
  - difficulty paying attention to what he or she is doing and trouble making choices

  A person with a history of serious depression before the illness is vulnerable to depression after a major life stress. A serious illness like cancer often triggers depression in these people. Professional help is usually required to help them.

- **You notice wide mood swings from periods of depression to periods of agitation and high energy.** Some people who have wide, uncontrollable swings in mood may have a "manic-depressive" illness. They cycle between being depressed with low energy and having a great deal of energy with feelings of agitation or feeling "high." The moods often don't seem connected to what is going on around the person. This requires professional help to determine if medication is necessary.

- **Nothing you do seems to help, even those strategies that have worked in the past.**

How to get professional help

Getting help for depression is just like getting help for physical problems. Asking for help doesn't mean you are saying the person is crazy. The problem could be caused by the stress related to cancer or by the treatment itself. Or it could be an understandable reaction to the serious issues a person with cancer must face.

Some people are hesitant to ask for professional help with their emotional problems because they are embarrassed. They may think seeing a psychologist, psychiatrist, or social worker means they are weak or strange. Being upset during a major illness is normal. So is getting help for these problems. Professionals such as social workers, nurse counselors, clergy, psychologists, and psychiatrists are skilled and experienced in helping people deal with emotionally stressful experiences. They are there to help you with this kind of problem—just like your family doctor is there to help with physical problems.

Ask for help from the physician who is treating the cancer, a family doctor, or another physician who is familiar with the medical treatments being given. Physicians familiar with the person's medical condition and treatments can evaluate whether the depression is due to the disease or the treatment. If it's due to the treatment, then a change in treatment may be needed. Physicians can also evaluate whether antidepression medications may help and can prescribe them if necessary. They can also make a referral to a mental health professional.

Ask a mental health professional such as a social worker, psychiatric or mental health nurse, psychologist, or psychiatrist for help. Mental health professionals are experienced in helping people with many types of emotional problems. They can be especially helpful when there is a history of depression before the illness and when the depression is not due to the person's disease or treatments. Many psychologists, social workers, and other mental health professionals have experience working with people with cancer. They can be very helpful when depression is a reaction to the stress of the illness. Many insurance plans require a referral from the primary care physician, so check on whether this is necessary.

Changing depressed feelings takes time. It usually takes at least several sessions with a counselor or therapist before a person begins to feel better. It also takes time for medicines to work, and the doctor may need to adjust the doses before the medicines are helpful.

What You Can Do to Help

Take care of your own emotional needs when caring for a depressed person

Many people are aware that depression happens frequently among persons with cancer. However, fewer people recognize that family members and friends who care for someone with cancer also often experience depression during the illness. All the stress can make a person feel "burned out." When someone feels this drained, he or she won't be much help to another person.

Caregiving can be stressful. To do your best in this difficult role, you need to find ways to stay emotionally well yourself. Here are some things that you can do for your own emotional health.

Understand that it is not your fault if the person becomes depressed. It is important to realize that you are not responsible if the person you are caring for becomes depressed. Depression can be caused by many things, including biological changes, treatment side effects, and changes in his or her life. Sometimes, especially if the depression is severe, only professionals can help. Do not feel guilty if, in spite of your best efforts, the person with cancer becomes or stays depressed.

Schedule positive experiences for yourself. Keep doing things that make you feel good. Don't become so involved in your caring responsibilities that you neglect your own emotional health. Don't feel guilty about taking care of yourself. If you become overwhelmed, you won't be able to provide care and support. You will be a better caregiver if you take time to do things you enjoy outside of your caring responsibilities. Do this early. This can help prevent your becoming seriously depressed and give you the strength to carry on. Social workers can help you arrange for care so you can take time off. Also, don't be afraid to ask family or friends to give care while you are away.

Get the companionship you need. Remember that you need companionship. Being with others is as important for you as for the person you are caring for. Continue to do things with people you like and enjoy. This helps to prevent and manage your own "blues." If you feel yourself becoming depressed, seek out other people to talk to and do things with. Some people find it helpful to talk to other people about their problems. If there is a support group for caregivers in your community, you can talk about your problems with others who understand your situation. Some people find it more helpful to talk about things that have nothing to do with their problems. This depends on how you feel and on the person you are talking to.

You can get professional help for yourself, too, if necessary.

Work as a team with the person who is depressed

Acknowledge the person is depressed. Don't ignore the person's depression. Sometimes people act as if the depression weren't there, either because they don't want to encourage it or because they don't want to deal with it. This is not healthy! It is uncomfortable to acknowledge someone you care for is depressed, but ignoring depression only makes it worse. The depressed person may feel you do not care.

Help before the depression becomes severe. If you ignore the early signs of depression, it is more likely to get out of hand, to seriously affect the quality of life of the person with cancer, and to require professional help.

Agree with positive thinking and correct those thoughts that seem wrong to you. Some of the depressed person's thoughts are correct. Make clear that you accept and agree with the correct parts. You are only disagreeing with the parts that seem wrong. You can point out, in a supportive way, the incorrect thoughts.

Practice giving helpful responses. A depressed person might say, "Nothing is going right." However, there is usually something that is going okay. You can say, "I understand you're feeling discouraged, but let's think of some of the things that are going right."

The depressed person might say, "I'm a total failure." However, you know that his or her whole life is not a failure. You might then say, "Maybe you've failed at some things, but think of all the things you have accomplished"—and then talk about several of them.

Encourage him or her to discuss the depression with a health professional who understands the treatments being received. See the discussion on asking for help from the physician who is treating the cancer on page 103.

Prevent or reduce depression

Much of the work here has to come from the person with cancer. In this section, we describe several ways to prevent or reduce depression. We recommend both you and the person with cancer read them carefully. If he or she cannot or does not want to read this plan, then explain the ideas and how you can help. These techniques work for most people. Your primary role is to be a team member by helping the person you are caring for learn these strategies and then by being supportive and encouraging their use.

Increase the number of activities that the person with cancer does with other people. Being with people you know and enjoy is an excellent way to take attention away from negative thoughts and feelings. It provides opportunities to think about one's own life in comparison to others and to recognize the good things in one's life. It provides opportunities to give as well as to receive help, to share experiences and perspectives, and to get help in dealing with problems that are making the person with cancer depressed. Most important is that other people can express caring and love for the person with cancer. Knowing other people care and are available to help when needed gives people strength and confidence when facing an uncertain future.

Make a list of friends and family members who have the following qualities:

- People who are sympathetic and understanding
- People who give good advice and who can help solve problems
- People who can turn attention away from problems and toward pleasant experiences

Think of how to make a visit pleasant and rewarding for them, and then reach out to them and ask for their help.

Encourage him or her to set reasonable, attainable goals. Depressed people tend to set goals that are too high, and when they don't reach their goals, they tend to become even more depressed. When you plan positive experiences, be sure that your goals are reasonable. It is better to set a low goal and accomplish more than you expected than to set too high a goal and fail. "Start low and go slow."

Make a plan to let the person with cancer know when you think he or she is doing things that may lead to depression. This helps him or her manage the depression early, before it becomes severe. Some people find it easiest to use a code word or phrase that the two of you agree on to point out depressed thinking. However you do it, a gentle reminder to stop and think about negative thoughts can help prevent the depression from setting in.

Support his or her efforts to control repetitive, negative thoughts and to substitute positive experiences and thoughts. When the person with cancer tells you that he or she needs to do something to "break out" of depressive thoughts, you can help by encouraging and becoming involved. This can be as simple as talking about something pleasant or doing an activity together.

Techniques for controlling negative thoughts

You can use this section to help the person with cancer control negative thoughts. You may want to suggest he or she read this section, or you may read it to the person with cancer and discuss it together.

THOUGHT STOPPING

One of the hard things about depression is that it's so easy to get stuck in a whirlwind of negative thinking. Suddenly you may find depressing thoughts going around and around in your head. It doesn't take long for this to make you feel bad, and then it may seem like you can't stop it. But you can!

The thought-stopping technique helps you "snap out of it" when that whirlwind of negative thoughts first starts. If you catch it early, you can keep it from getting you too upset. The trick is to do this when you first notice a negative thought.

When you first feel yourself in the negative-thinking whirlwind, try one of these techniques:

- **Yell "STOP!" really loudly in your mind.** When you scream STOP in your mind, pretend it is very loud. The idea is to wake you up, to make you aware that you're in danger of getting stuck in negative thoughts. You might start this by going to a place by yourself and shouting STOP out loud. Practice it this way until you can do it in your mind alone.

  Visualize a big red STOP sign. Try to see it clearly, and then get your mind on something else. Think of what a STOP sign looks like. Make sure you see it as a red sign. Practice seeing it in your mind so you can bring it to mind easily. Now whenever you catch yourself starting negative thoughts, think of this image and stop yourself.

- **Slap yourself on the wrist with a rubber band.** Another way to remind yourself to stop is to gently slap your wrist with a rubber band. This isn't to punish yourself. This is to give you a physical reminder to stop the thoughts.
- **Splash some water on your face.** Splashing water in your face is another way to wake yourself up from the negative thinking. Pay attention to how the water makes you feel.
- **Get up and move to a new spot.** Getting up and moving to a new spot gives you a change of scenery. You can use the new surroundings to help you think about other things.
- **Start some pleasant, involving activity** that takes all your attention and pushes out the negative thinking.
- **Fight the negative thoughts.** Maybe several of these techniques together will work for you.
- **Arrange a time and a place for negative thinking.** This technique allows you to think about negative things, but puts you in control of when and where you do this thinking.
- **Find a negative-thinking "office."** This can be a room, a chair, or just a certain window. Make this the only place you let yourself think about all of the negative things.

  Your "office" space can be any place you choose. Don't, however, make it your bed or where you eat. These need to be "safe zones." Now try to only think your negative thoughts in this one place.
- **Write down your negative thoughts on a piece of paper.** This can help you to see them in perspective. Then rip the paper into small pieces and throw it away.
- **Schedule a time each day when you plan to think your negative thoughts.** Scheduling a time to think about your negative

thoughts helps you to take control of them. You might not be able to control all negative thinking, especially in the beginning, but this technique will gradually help you to get control over your negative thinking.

Don't make this time around mealtimes, just before you go to sleep, or just before you expect to see people. These should be relaxing times. Make this time no more that 15 minutes. At the end of 15 minutes, stop. You can continue tomorrow.

When you're depressed, you may look at techniques for stopping these thoughts and say, "That's silly. It could never work." Actually, research has shown that they can work. Give them a try!

DISTRACTION

You can't think about two things at once. When you start thinking negative thoughts, get your mind involved in another activity that "pushes out" or replaces the negative thinking. Try one of these ideas:

- Take a vacation in your mind. Close your eyes and think about your favorite spot. Spend a couple minutes there on a mental vacation. Relax and enjoy it.

- Mentally time travel into the future. Think of something you are looking forward to. Imagine it is happening. Think of how nice it is to be there.

  When you take your mental vacation or time travel to something you're looking forward to, really try to work your imagination. Think about as many details as possible. Here are some suggestions:

  - What does it feel like? Is there a warm breeze? Imagine how it feels on your skin.

  - What does it sound like? Are there waves gently crashing on the beach? Are people laughing, or is music playing? Imagine it as clearly and vividly as you can.

  - What does it look like? Is the sky clear and blue? Or are you in a room? Imagine what the room looks like. Try to see it as completely as you can.

- What does it smell like? Is it the salty smell of the ocean? Maybe you smell the fragrances of a garden or a big dinner.
- What does it taste like? Are you drinking a nice cool drink? Feel it in your mouth. Taste it.

Use these exercises to fill your mind with as many pleasant details as you can. Think of as many as you can. This exercise is also helpful when you are feeling anxious and need help falling asleep.

TENSION BUSTING

Use the relaxation exercises on pages 98–99. Being relaxed helps you to think about pleasant things.

DO SOMETHING YOU LIKE

Really get yourself involved in an activity you like. This will push out bad thoughts. The idea of this exercise is to fill your mind up with positive thoughts and to have them crowd out the negative ones.

ARGUING AGAINST NEGATIVE THOUGHTS

The idea of this exercise is to make yourself see both sides of the picture. Things aren't usually as bad as they first seem when you're depressed. However, the only way to see the other side is to actively argue against it.

You can fight your negative thoughts. Challenge their accuracy. Every situation has at least two sides to it. When you're depressed, you probably only see the bad side. If you weren't depressed, you would usually think of both sides. This exercise forces you to actively take the other side. It is like having a debate with yourself.

- Begin by asking yourself, "Is your negative thought really true?" Make yourself be clear about what evidence supports it.
- Now take the other side. Argue the exact opposite. Think of every reason why your thought may not be true or may be exaggerated. Don't give up too easily. Really argue as if you were arguing with someone else.
- When you're arguing with your negative thoughts, try to be as complete as possible. You may want to write down the answers to the following questions:
  - What is the evidence against my negative thought?

- Are there any "facts" in my thinking that are really just assumptions?
- Is my argument an example of "black and white" thinking? Are there shades of gray that I'm ignoring?
- Is the negative side taking things out of context? Am I looking at the whole picture or just one small part of it?
- Am I trying to predict the future when I really know that I can't?

- Try to punch as many holes in your "negative sides" argument as you can. Don't accept any illogical thinking at all.
- Solve day-to-day problems that are causing you stress
- Use a problem-solving approach to solving some of the day-to-day problems that are contributing to your feelings of depression, such as finding enough time to do housework, problems with family members, and so on.

Possible Obstacles

Here are some obstacles that other people have faced in helping a person with cancer deal with depression:

"I don't want your help. Leave me alone."

"I can't do anything without your cooperation. You must participate in the plan if it is going to be effective. I will not do anything without your agreement and cooperation. We have to start small—with something that is easy to do—and then evaluate the results. If your depression is so severe that you don't even want to try, then we should get professional help."

"My problems are real! It's normal to be depressed in my situation."

"Your problems are real and some sadness is normal. However, getting stuck in the feeling of depression can interfere with dealing with the problems that are causing the depression. The goal is to keep a balance between positive and negative thoughts. The problems are real, but many of the good things in life are also real and should get equal attention."

"Nothing will help, so it's no use trying."

"That's the depression talking—not you. Give it a try! There is nothing to lose and a good deal to gain. We'll start with small, manageable things that are easy to do and then we can decide if these ideas are helpful. If you are so depressed that you can't even try, then we need to get professional help."

Think of other obstacles that could interfere with carrying out your plan

What additional roadblocks could get in the way of doing the things recommended in this chapter? For example, will the person with cancer cooperate? Will other people help? Do you have the time and energy to carry out the plan?

Develop plans for getting around these roadblocks using the six problem-solving steps discussed in the first section of this book (see pages xi–xvi).

Carrying Out and Adjusting Your Plan

Carrying out your plan

Talk this plan over with the person with cancer. Agree together on what you can do together to manage depression. It is important to work as a team when dealing with these problems. Sometimes the support and the feeling of being on a team is in itself helpful to a depressed person.

Use these techniques early. Look for beginning signs of depression and put your plan into action then—don't wait until depression is severe. The techniques discussed in this plan have helped severely depressed persons, but usually as part of professional treatment. As a caregiver, you can help most before depression becomes severe.

Plan in advance what you will do to manage depression. If you know the person with cancer is likely to be depressed at certain times based on past experience, then make plans for what you will do to prevent depression from building up.

Persist. Even if the person with cancer continues to feel depressed, don't give up. You are probably preventing the depression from getting worse. Keep working cooperatively with the depressed person. If you are working together, these ideas can only help.

Checking on results

Talk regularly with the person with cancer about his or her feelings. Although it may be difficult for you at first, let the person with cancer know you understand depression can happen during this illness. If you show you are comfortable talking about feelings, the person with cancer is more likely to let you know early on if he or she is experiencing depressive symptoms.

It may seem scary at first to talk to a depressed person about what is upsetting him or her. However, it's important to do this because it shows you care, and it helps you work together, as a team, to control the depressed thoughts and feelings.

Watch for indications that professional help is needed.

If your plan doesn't work...

Ask if you are expecting change too fast. It usually takes time to manage depression. Look for a small improvement at first. Remember: Your efforts may be successful even if they just keep the depression from getting worse.

If these techniques do not seem to be helping and the person with cancer has been feeling very depressed for several weeks, review this chapter to be sure you have tried all of the ideas. If so, encourage the person with cancer to seek professional help.

CAREGIVING

Physical Conditions

This section is particularly helpful to caregivers because it addresses common physical conditions that people with cancer face. The chapters include *Appetite, Bleeding, Cancer Pain, Confusion and Seizures, Constipation, Diarrhea, Fever and Infections, Mouth Conditions, Nausea and Vomiting, Skin Conditions,* and *Vein Conditions (Needle Sticks).*

The information in this section fits most situations, but yours may be different. If the doctor or nurse tells you to do something else, follow what they say. If you think there may be a medical emergency, see the *When to Get Professional Help* section of each chapter.

This section explains conditions that many people with cancer face. Encourage the person with cancer to read this information, and then you can work together as a team.

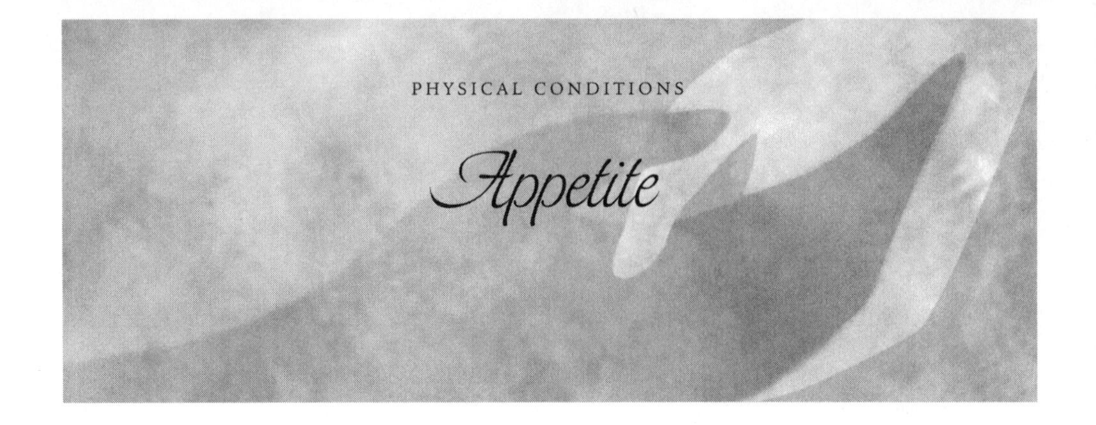

Understanding the Condition

Preparing and serving food is often an important part of caregiving. It is a very personal way to show we care. How well a person who is ill eats is an indication of his or her health. So it is natural to pay a lot of attention to how a person with cancer eats. However, it's important not to focus too much on eating. This can make the person with cancer upset, which can actually decrease his or her appetite. It's best to take a relaxed, positive attitude toward eating. This chapter lists many things you can do to help the person's appetite and to increase the amount of nutritious food consumed.

People with cancer may lose their appetite for many reasons. Cancer treatments and other medicines can decrease the desire for food, as can emotional distress or worry.

Losing weight can upset the person with cancer especially if he or she sees it as a sign the illness is getting worse. Rapid weight loss can often be slowed down by stopping diarrhea, giving high-calorie foods, or taking medicines prescribed to increase appetite.

This chapter lists things you can do to increase appetite.

Your goals are to:

- call for professional help when it is needed
- help increase appetite
- cover up tastes and smells that are bothersome
- prevent an early feeling of fullness
- add more proteins and calories to food
- be able to help in care of gastrointestinal (GI) feeding tubes if they are used
- encourage healthy eating

When to Get Professional Help

Call the doctor or nurse if any of the following conditions exist:

- ▲ **The person has had very little to eat or drink in one or more days.** Ask the doctor or nurse when to report a poor appetite. If nausea causes the loss of appetite, then read the chapter *Nausea and Vomiting* (pages 202–210) for steps you can take to relieve that symptom. When nausea lasts more than a few days and little is eaten, it's important to keep the doctor or nurse informed so the situation doesn't develop into an emergency.
- ▲ **Five pounds are lost in one week.** Ask the doctor or nurse when to call about weight loss. If the person with cancer is losing weight, then talk about this on a clinic visit or with the home health nurse if one is visiting the home.
- ▲ **There is pain with chewing or swallowing.** Painful chewing or swallowing interferes with normal eating and drinking. Pain can be caused by a mouth sore or an infection on the tongue, gums, or throat. If the appetite suddenly changes, ask the person if he or she is having trouble eating, chewing, or swallowing.

(The underlined numbers above should be used as a general guide. Check with your doctor or nurse for information specific to your situation.)

Know the following facts before you call the doctor or nurse:

- When did the poor appetite problem start? ________________
- How much weight has been lost? ________________________
- Has this problem happened before? If so, what brought the appetite back or helped it improve? ______________________
- Does food taste differently, for example, bitter or metallic? If so, does this make foods less desirable? ______________________
- Which foods taste better and which taste worse than they used to?

  ____

  ____
- Is the person's mouth dry or sore and is swallowing difficult?

  ____

- Does he or she have medicine to help with mouth problems? If so, what is the brand and dose? ____________________________
- Does the person feel full or bloated soon after starting to eat? ____
- Is the person having nausea, vomiting, or problems with bowels such as constipation or diarrhea? If so, what medicines are available in the home for these problems and which of these have they tried for this problem?____________________________
- When the appetite changed, was there a change in where or how food was eaten? ____________________________
- Does the person have a better or worse appetite at certain meals or at certain times of day? ____________________________

Here is an example of what you might say when calling for help:

"My husband is Dr. Lipton's patient. His mouth is so sore that he's having trouble chewing."

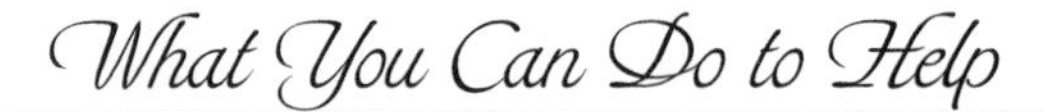

There are several things you can do to manage appetite problems:

- help increase the appetite
- cover up tastes or smells that are bothersome
- prevent an early feeling of fullness
- add more protein and calories to food
- help in the care of GI feeding tubes if used
- encourage healthy eating

Help increase the appetite

There are several things you can do that will help stimulate appetite.

Encourage light exercise or walking before meals, in fresh air if possible. Any increase in activity just before eating increases the appetite. Suggest walking five to fifteen minutes up to half an hour before meals.

Serve meals with other people, whenever possible. Avoid eating alone. Eating with someone else is distracting and can increase the amount a person eats by taking attention away from food. Sometimes meal habits change after a diagnosis of cancer because the family schedule is disrupted by trips to clinics for checkups and treatments. Returning to normal meal times and planning to have the family eat together helps to increase the appetite.

Serve meals in a pleasant, relaxed atmosphere, if possible.

Use small plates and serve smaller portions. A small portion on a small plate can be arranged attractively and looks like something that can be finished.

Keep food out of sight when not eating. Keep food off countertops and put it in containers you can't see through. Then the person with cancer is not reminded about the appetite problem by seeing food all of the time and food may be more appealing when served.

Serve lemonade or orange juice only if the mouth is not sore. Juices contain acids that can stimulate appetites. Four ounces of juice before a meal may improve the appetite.

Serve a glass of wine, a beer, or a cocktail before lunch or dinner, if the doctor approves. Alcohol stimulates the appetite. However, alcohol should not be taken with certain medicines and should not be taken before chemotherapy treatments because it can cause nausea and even change the effect of the drugs. Ask the doctor and pharmacist about alcohol limits or about drinking alcohol at all.

Minimize or eliminate tastes and smells that are bothersome

Cancer treatments frequently change how foods taste. There are a number of things you can do to make food appealing again.

Use plastic instead of metal utensils. Plastic does not add a bitter or metal taste, which is a common complaint among persons receiving chemotherapy.

Try new spices, such as basil, curry, coriander, mint, oregano, or rosemary. Spices make our mouths water and change the tastes of food. You may find a new spice that makes the person hungry again. Try old spices in new ways because the chemotherapy sometimes changes the way food tastes.

Add new flavors, such as lemon, beer, pickles, salad dressings, vinegar, mayonnaise, relishes, fruit juices, or wines.

Marinate meats in liquids, such as fruit juices, salad dressings, wine, sweet and sour sauce, soy sauce, or barbecue sauce. Sauces and marinades change the flavor of food and make it more appealing.

Sprinkle more sugar and salt in food if these are not restricted. These decrease the metal and bitter tastes that persons with cancer sometimes complain about. Some people receiving chemotherapy cannot tolerate a sweet taste, in which case they use smaller amounts of sugar than before.

Serve carbohydrates and high-protein foods. High protein foods include fish, chicken, meat, turkey, eggs, cheeses, milk, ice cream, tofu, nuts, peanut butter, yogurt, beans, or peas. Foods high in carbohydrates include bread, pasta, and potatoes. Try to get as much protein and as many carbohydrates as possible in each food item served. This is called "power-packing."

Serve food cold. A cold temperature downplays the smell and taste of food. Aromas are blocked or linger for shorter times, and cold foods are not as flavorful, so odd tastes are covered up. Also, the coolness numbs the tongue to some unpleasant tastes.

Encourage sucking on hard, sugar-free, sour, or mint candy. These candies can mask strange tastes any time of the day and before a meal. These may also help with nausea and vomiting if that is a problem.

Offer ginger ale or mint tea. They cover up metallic tastes and help with swallowing food.

Avoid most red meats and serve chicken, fish, or pork. Changes in the taste buds may make red meat distasteful. People receiving chemotherapy often prefer chicken or fish.

Prevent an early feeling of fullness

Poor appetite can be caused by an early feeling of being full. Sometimes medicines cause gas, and the person feels bloated after eating just a little bit. Here are several things that can be done to help.

Exercise between meals. Any exercise gets the intestinal tract moving and shakes up pockets of gas. Even stretching and bending at the waist when getting out of chairs or off of couches helps relieve gas and move stomach contents downward.

Walk around or sit up for awhile after meals, but avoid strenuous exercise immediately after eating. Walking or sitting up helps to empty the stomach and break up any gas that adds to a sense of fullness and discomfort.

Drink beverages between meals instead of with meals. Liquids at mealtime can make the stomach feel full. Drinking less while eating allows more room for food.

Eat small amounts of food six to eight times a day. Small, frequent meals or snacks prevent an early sense of fullness, and more food can be eaten over a 24-hour period.

Eat slowly and chew food well.

Avoid certain vegetables and carbonation. Cut back on fatty foods and gas-producing foods such as beans, cucumbers, green peppers, onions, broccoli, brussels sprouts, corn, cauliflower, sauerkraut, turnips, cabbage, chewing gum, milk, rutabagas, or carbonated beverages. Some vegetables are digested slowly or create stomach and intestinal gas, which causes a feeling of fullness. Avoid carbonated sodas or waters that can make the stomach feel full when it isn't. Remove the carbonation by opening cans and bottles early and letting the fizz evaporate and the sodas turn flat.

Use over-the-counter medicines (that can be bought without a prescription) to help break up gas. Many of these medicines contain herbs or drugs that break up gas. One particular ingredient, simethicone, is helpful in attacking gas and breaking up air trapped in the intestines. Check with the doctor and nurse before buying these over-the-counter medicines because they shouldn't be used with some other medicines.

Add proteins and calories to diet

Rapid weight loss can often be slowed by increasing the nutritional value of food that is eaten, especially by increasing the calories and proteins. Here are some suggestions for how you can prepare and serve foods.

Offer small, frequent snacks (six per day) even if the person is not hungry, and encourage eating as much as wanted. Smaller meals and snacks may result in more food intake than three large meals.

Add butter or margarine to vegetables, soups, pasta, cooked cereal, and rice. These add fat and calories and improve the taste of many foods.

Add sugar, syrup, honey, and jelly to vegetables, meats, cereals, waffles, and rolls. Sweet sauces add calories and can make dry foods easier to swallow.

Use sour cream, cream cheese, ricotta cheese, or yogurt on baked potatoes, vegetables, and crackers. Creams are fattening, nutritious, and easy to swallow.

Add whipped cream to hot chocolate, ice cream, pies, puddings, gelatin, and other desserts. Whipped cream is loaded with calories and has a pleasant taste. Add sugar to whipped cream and boost calories even higher.

Add powdered coffee creamers or powdered milk to gravy, sauces, soups, and hot cereals. These are good sources of calcium and increase the number of calories in food without adding bulk.

Use milk, soy milk, or plain yogurt instead of water to dilute condensed soups or cooked cereals. If a recipe calls for water, use these milk products instead. This will add calories and important nutrients and vitamins.

Use mayonnaise instead of salad dressing and use light cream instead of milk in recipes. Mayonnaise and light cream have more fat and calories than salad dressing and milk. Avoid skim milk, if possible.

Add ice cream, tofu, ricotta cheese, or yogurt to milk drinks. These products increase the fat and calorie content in milk drinks and feel good on sore throats. Mix them well in a blender.

Add one cup of nonfat dry milk to one quart of whole milk for drinking and cooking. You can more than double the protein and calorie content of whole milk if you add powdered dry milk to it.

Use half-and-half or evaporated milk instead of water in recipes. Half cream and half milk or evaporated milk are much higher in fat, protein, and calories. They also provide vital minerals and nutrients. Drinking instant breakfast mixes, which are sold in grocery stores, is another way to get extra calories.

Use peanut butter on crackers, bread, waffles, apple wedges, or celery sticks. Peanut butter is an excellent source of protein.

Offer crushed granola, nuts, seeds, or wheat germ in shakes or on desserts. Nuts are a great snack between meals.

Use commercial nutritional supplements or your own milkshakes between meals or with snacks. These powders or liquids are loaded with nutrients and can be purchased in most drug stores. Ask the nurse or pharmacist for information about specific products and ask for recipes.

Avoid diets designed to "purge the system." Certain diets are designed to purge or empty the intestinal tract. Unfortunately, they also remove important vitamins, minerals, and fluids from the body. The person with cancer needs these nutrients.

Ask the nurse or doctor about using vitamin supplements and iron. Vitamin supplements replace some vitamins lost because of a smaller appetite and smaller intake of food. The doctor or nurse may suggest daily multivitamin and iron pills as supplements to the diet.

Help with care of GI tubes and feedings if used

If the person cannot swallow food, GI tubes are sometimes used to put food into the stomach. They may be used after surgery and are temporary until healing occurs. They can also be permanent. GI tubes are inserted into a hole that goes directly into the intestinal tract. A few times a day the tube is unclamped and connected to a bag holding a thick nutritious fluid and the fluid drips into the tube.

Ask the nurse to show you how to care for skin around the GI tube and how to give a tube feeding. You can ask for a home visit from a nurse to help you solve problems with this kind of feeding and to teach you how to do it yourself.

Encourage healthy eating

Good nutrition is important for people with cancer. Eating well helps them cope with the side effects of treatment. Healthy eating helps to keep up strength, build immune system functioning, rebuild tissues, and speed healing.

Offer a variety of foods, including:

- fruits and vegetables, which provide important vitamins such as A and C as well as minerals the body needs. Five or more servings of any combination each day is a good guideline.
- protein, which helps tissues heal and fight infection. Examples are fish, chicken, meat, eggs, and cheese. Three or more servings each day is a good guideline.
- grains, which provide carbohydrates and B vitamins. Grains are a good source of energy. Examples are bread, pasta, and cereals. Try to eat three to five servings each day.
- dairy foods, which are an important source of protein, calcium, and many vitamins. Examples include yogurt, ice cream, cheese, and other milk products. Two to three servings each day is a good guideline.

Possible Obstacles

Here are some obstacles that other caregivers have faced when trying to solve appetite problems:

"He says he's just not interested in food. He's not hungry at all."

Lack of interest in food cannot be easily changed. Try offering small snacks or meals in the company of people he or she enjoys. Try the other suggestions in this chapter, but don't focus on eating so much so that it's the only topic you ask about or talk about. Constantly talking about needing to eat may turn off the person's appetite.

"Why bother with adding calories to food? The treatments make her so nauseated that she won't eat anyway."

Cancer treatments do not cause as much nausea as they used to. New drugs to prevent nausea are very good now. Adding calories to food helps to prevent anemia and increase energy. It will also help keep weight on. All of these benefits help the person with cancer handle the cancer treatments and feel better.

Think of other obstacles that could interfere with carrying out your plan

What additional roadblocks could get in the way of doing the things recommended in this chapter? For example, will the person with cancer cooperate? Will other people help? How will you explain your needs to other people? Do you have the time and energy to carry out the plan?

Develop plans for getting around these roadblocks using the six problem-solving steps discussed in the first section of this book (see pages xi–xvi).

Carrying Out and Adjusting Your Plan

Checking on results

Keep track of the amount of food the person with cancer is eating as well as his or her weight. If you find a problem, check this chapter on whether to call the doctor or nurse. Ask if eating is being hindered by bothersome tastes and smells, dry or sore mouth, or an early feeling of fullness. If so, use the ideas in this chapter.

If your plan doesn't work...

If you are not satisfied with progress about eating, talk about your concerns with the doctor or nurse. They may refer you to a dietician who will give you new ideas or tell you whether the diet is adequate and whether you are packing as many nutrients as you can into the foods you are serving. The doctor may also prescribe an appetite stimulant or make other suggestions to help you deal with this problem.

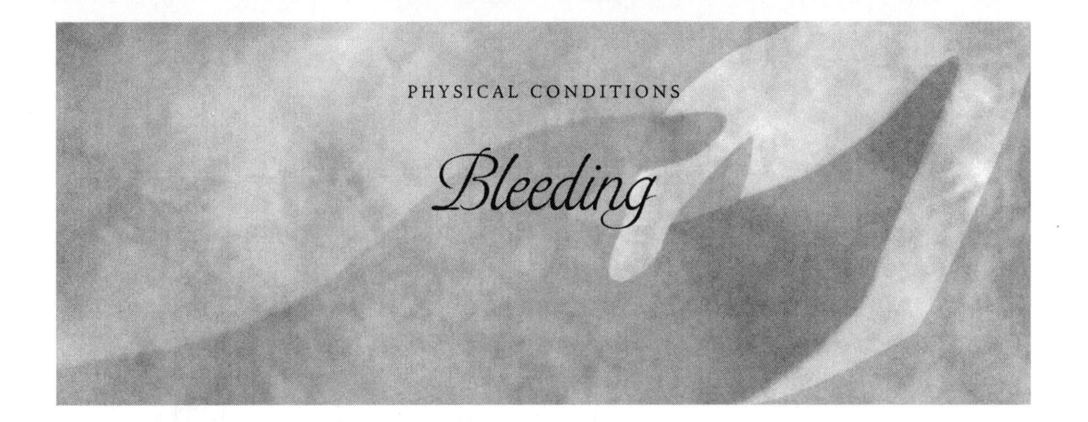

PHYSICAL CONDITIONS

Bleeding

Understanding the Condition

This is a good chapter to read in advance so that you are prepared if bleeding or bruising happens to the person you are caring for. Sometimes you will need to act quickly to get medical help. Sometimes you will have to deal with the bleeding yourself until you get medical advice or help. There are also things you can do to reduce the chances that bleeding or bruising will happen.

People receiving certain kinds of chemotherapy are at higher risk for unusual bleeding, such as after shaving or brushing their teeth. This is because chemotherapy affects the bone marrow's ability to make platelets, and the number of platelets drops after certain kinds of chemotherapy. Platelets are made inside the bone marrow and help the blood to clot, or stop flowing. Sometimes the doctor will prescribe medicines that increase the growth of platelets.

When a person is receiving chemotherapy, ask whether it affects bleeding. If it does, ask when to get professional help if bleeding occurs, how to spot bleeding in its early stages, how to control bleeding, and how to help prevent it.

Platelets

Your goals are to:

- call when professional help is needed
- prevent bleeding
- identify bleeding in its early stages if possible
- control bleeding if it starts

When to Get Professional Help

Urge the person with cancer to call the doctor or nurse or make the call yourself if any of the following conditions exist:

- **Any unusual or sudden bleeding lasting more than 10 minutes, such as nose bleeds or bleeding gums.** Tiny capillaries at the end of the blood flow system branch out through the whole body. Most bleeding that we can see comes from these small blood vessels. The nose and mouth have many of these capillaries near the surface of the skin. These are the easiest places to break open and bleed.

- **Vomiting of blood or coffee ground-type material.** In rare cases, bright red blood can be vomited. Blood in vomit, however, is more likely to be very dark in color and look like coffee grounds. This is blood that has been collecting in the stomach or abdomen because of a bleeding ulcer or sore.

- **Blood in the urine.** Look for red, pink, or dark urine. Urine is usually light yellow. It is a darker yellow when it is more concentrated, for example, when a person is not drinking much fluid. Pink or red urine indicates a problem with bleeding. A change from yellow to a dark-colored urine should also be reported, although it may not be caused by blood.

- **Blood in the stool.** Look for red, dark red, or black stools. Bright red blood around a stool means blood vessels close to the rectum are open and bleeding. Hemorrhoids can cause this. Dark black or tar-colored stools indicate a bleeding problem higher in the intestinal tract since the blood is older and darker by the time it comes out in the stool.

- **Tiny red spots on the skin (or in the mouth) or bruising, either of which appear quickly and without any apparent cause.** Tiny capillaries or blood vessels can open up in areas where they are closest to the skin surface. When they bleed underneath the skin, they leave dots or spots that are red or purple.

- **Cough, sputum, or phlegm with blood.** Very small amounts of blood or streaks of blood may appear when the person with cancer coughs up phlegm (a thick, wet discharge produced after coughing). If this happens more than once or if the phlegm is quite bloody, report it to the doctor.

Know the following facts before you call the doctor or nurse:

- When did this sign of bleeding start? ____________________
- How long did it last? ____________________
- How much was there? ____________________
- Has the person coughed up blood? ____________________
- For women: Is there vaginal bleeding? How heavy is the flow?

  ____
- Is there bleeding anywhere else? Where? ____________________
- What medicines were taken recently? At what dosage?
  - Aspirin ____________________
  - Ibuprofen, Motrin, Advil ____________________
  - Alka Seltzer ____________________
  - Iron ____________________
  - Suppositories ____________________
  - Chemotherapy (when?) ____________________

    ____ Prednisone

    ____ Decadron
  - Nasal sprays ____________________
  - Sinus medicines ____________________
  - Arthritis medicines ____________________
  - Herbal medicines or supplements ____________________
  - Other medicines (explain what they are) ____________________

    ____
- Is the person receiving radiation therapy? If yes, where on the body and how recently? ____________________
- Has the person received chemotherapy recently? If yes, what was the chemotherapy and when was it received? ____________________
- Did the person with cancer have problems in the past with stomach ulcers or other bleeding problems? ____________________

- When were the last blood counts done, and what were the platelet levels? ______________________

Here's an example of what you might say when calling:

"My son sees Dr. Wilson at the oncology clinic. He just started chemotherapy this week and had a bad nosebleed. I was worried that the chemotherapy may have caused it."

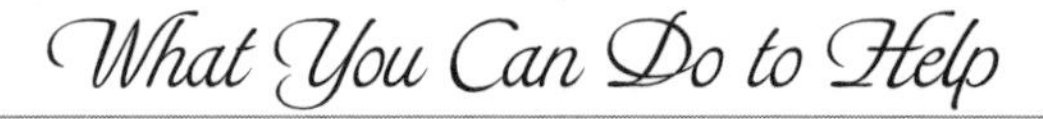

What You Can Do to Help

If the bleeding problem is not an emergency, there are some things you can do:

- control the bleeding
- prevent future bleeding

Control the bleeding

When bleeding starts, it often flows from tiny capillaries that are near the skin surface, such as from the nose or gums. These capillaries open easily, but they also close easily. Try the following three methods to stop the bleeding:

Press on the area of bleeding. Pressing on the skin gives the blood in the capillaries more time to clot. Apply pressure to the skin around the bleeding site for about four minutes using a clean, dry washcloth to maintain the pressure. Do not look to see if the bleeding has stopped until after four minutes. You can also use an elastic bandage or gauze and firmly tape it around the wound, depending on where the bleeding is.

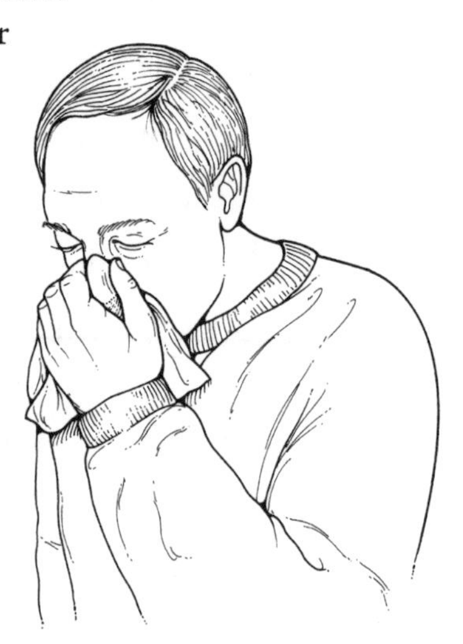

For nosebleeds, put ice on the nose and press the nose and back of the neck with your hand. Pressing gives more time to stop the bleeding. For a nosebleed, press the nostrils with a handkerchief or put ice wrapped in a soft cloth over the bridge of the nose for a full five minutes and press firmly on the nostrils. Ice makes the capillaries shrink, which helps to control bleeding. Do not check to see if the bleeding has stopped or look at the nosebleed until after five minutes have gone by.

Tilt head forward slightly for nosebleeds, but don't lie down because this causes blood to drip into the throat. Try not to swallow the blood during a nosebleed since swallowed blood can cause nausea and vomiting.

NOTE: The following section can be used to help prevent bleeding if platelet counts are low due to chemotherapy. **These methods are not meant to be used regularly.** Check with your doctor or nurse if you have questions.

Prevent bleeding

There are many ways to prevent bleeding and bruising when the platelet count is low.

Do not use ibuprofen or ibuprofen products unless approved by your doctor. These include products such as Motrin, Advil, Naprosyn, Indocin, Anaprox, Clinoril, Feldene, or Tolestin. These drugs prevent the blood from clotting in the normal amount of time. Avoid giving these when platelet counts are low.

Do not use aspirin or products containing aspirin (ASA, acetylsalicylic acid, or salicylate) unless approved by your doctor. These include products such as Alka Seltzer, Dristan, Percodan, Anacin, Ecotrin, Pepto-Bismol, Ascriptin, Excedrin, Sominex, Bromoseltzer, Fiorinol, Vanquish, Congespirin, or Midol. At the drugstore, read the fine print on the label of any analgesic or pain relief pill (see *Appendix* on page 270). It may list aspirin or acetylsalicylic acid as one of the ingredients. This means the pill has aspirin in it. Aspirin makes a person bleed more easily, especially when platelet counts are low. Check with the pharmacist if you are not sure about a product.

Give aspirin-free products such as acetaminophen, Tylenol, Datril, or Aspirin-Free Anacin.

Do not floss teeth. This can cut the gums and bleeding may be hard to stop.

Buy soft toothbrushes or sponge-type toothbrushes. Gums bleed easily when irritated or scraped. A soft toothbrush treats the gums much more gently so that they are less likely to bleed.

Encourage rinsing and brushing teeth after eating. Rinsing helps remove left-over food, which can build up and start an abscess or sore and make the gums bleed. Avoid mouth washes with alcohol if the mouth is sore since they can burn the mouth.

Serve a soft, bland diet, such as soup, pureed meats, mashed potatoes, custards, gelatin, or puddings, if there is mouth soreness. Soft foods are the least likely to create a cut or scrape in the mouth. Bland, nonspicy foods are also less likely to cause bleeding. Avoid hot-temperature foods. Think back to when you burned the top of your mouth on pizza or a grilled cheese sandwich. The skin tore. When the platelets are low, the skin will also bleed if it tears because it was burnt.

Suggest using petroleum jelly or lip balm to keep lips moist and to prevent cracking.

Remind the person with cancer to blow the nose gently. There are many tiny blood vessels in and near the nose that can open up if the nose is blown too forcefully. Nasal sprays can cause nose bleeds if they are over-used or are too strong.

Encourage shaving only with an electric razor. Women can use hair removal products such as Nair or Neet.

Limit the use of sharp objects such as razors, knives, scissors, or tools.

Remind the person to avoid situations of potential harm and injury. When platelet counts are low, it's important to do things with as little risk of injury as possible. For example, take a car or bus rather than ride a bicycle or motorcycle. Avoid contact sports. It's easy for small blood vessels to be damaged by bumps or falls.

Ask others to do heavy lifting and strenuous activities.

Take steps to avoid constipation. Straining to move the bowels can cause bleeding, especially around the rectum. See the chapter *Constipation* (pages 165–173) for more explanation of what to do to avoid constipation.

Pad the top of the hands with gauze if bumping them is likely to happen. If bumping the hands happens a lot and bruising occurs, consider taping a small piece of gauze onto the top of the hands as protection. Padding reduces the chance of bruising a vein and opening it up to bleed.

Do not use rectal thermometers, suppositories, or enemas, or have rectal intercourse. Anything put into the rectum can tear these delicate tissues, and bleeding can start easily. Rectal intercourse can also cause bleeding.

Remind women with cancer not to use vaginal douches.

Keep open cuts or scrapes clean to avoid infection.

Learn about blood counts. Ask the staff to explain platelet counts, what makes them go up and down, and what happens to a person with cancer as platelet counts rise and fall.

Possible Obstacles

Here is one obstacle that other people have faced:

"I need to take aspirin for my arthritis."

Many arthritis medicines put the person with cancer at risk for bleeding, but at the same time they can help control pain. If you have a history of bleeding problems, then the risk of bleeding is greater. If pain control is important, this may override the risk. This is a decision you should make with your doctor—and not alone. You can ask your doctor about ways to control arthritis pain that do not increase the risk of bleeding.

Think of other obstacles that could interfere with carrying out your plan

What additional roadblocks could get in the way of doing the things recommended in this chapter? For example, will the person with cancer cooperate? Will other people help? How will you explain your needs to medical staff? Do you have the time and energy to carry out the plan?

Develop plans for getting around these roadblocks using the six problem-solving steps discussed in the first section of this book (see pages xi–xvi).

Carrying Out and Adjusting Your Plan

Checking on results

Are you getting professional help when it is needed? Are you able to stop the bleeding on your own whenever it starts? Are the skin and mouth as well cared for and protected as they can be? Are other precautions to prevent bleeding being followed?

Keep a close eye on this situation in case it changes. Keep track of blood counts and chemotherapy dates to know when the risk for bleeding is higher.

If your plan doesn't work...

If problems with bleeding are getting worse, then ask yourself if you are doing everything you can to protect the skin against bruises, bumps, or cuts and to encourage good oral hygiene. Also, review *When to Get Professional Help* (pages 128–130). If you call the doctor or nurse, report the facts about the bleeding (see pages 129–130) and what you have done to deal with the problem.

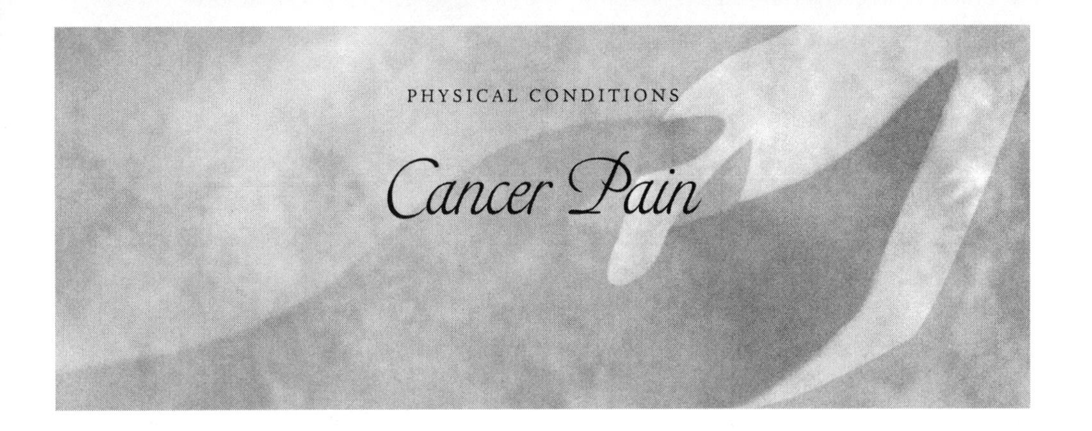

Understanding the Condition

As a family caregiver, you play a crucial role in managing cancer pain. You are often the one who gives pain medicines and who makes sure the health professionals are informed about and responsive to the person's pain. This is a long chapter with a lot of information, but we want you to have a good understanding of what can be done to control pain. Then you will know what questions to ask and be able to judge if the pain relief is the best possible.

Here are three key ideas to keep in mind as a family caregiver of someone with cancer pain:

1. Most cancer pain can be relieved, and all cancer pain can be controlled.
2. Every person with cancer has the right to the best pain control. Your job, as a home caregiver, is to be sure this happens.
3. It takes time to get good pain control, so have patience. On the other hand, do not give up until adequate pain control is achieved.

When many people think of cancer, they think of pain. However, today most cancer pain can be relieved. For example, even in cases of advanced cancer, pain has been controlled in 90 to 99 percent of those persons who are helped by health professionals who are experienced and knowledgeable about controlling pain. In nine of ten cases, cancer pain can be controlled by using pills alone. In those few situations in which pain cannot be relieved, it can be reduced so that the person with cancer can live with it day to day and accomplish activities important to him or her.

It is important that everyone be open and supportive about controlling pain. Family and friends need to make clear they believe the person's reports of pain. People with pain are the only people who know how much pain they are feeling. If people with pain feel others do not believe them, they become upset and may stop reporting their pain accurately. This only makes controlling the pain more difficult.

Pain medicines must be adjusted to each person's pain–which takes time. The doctor may have to try different medicines or amounts to see what works best. Do not give up just because complete pain control does not happen immediately. Keep in mind most cancer pain can eventually be relieved.

Pain is not always caused by a tumor. Many things can cause new aches and pains in addition to the growth of cancer itself. When people with pain feel something new, many think, "It is the cancer growing. This is a bad sign." However, the pain might not be from the cancer at all. For example, treatments cause tissues to shrink and swell and this can cause pain. Weight loss or gain also changes tissues and muscles, which may cause pain.

How health professionals control cancer pain

Doctors and other health professionals who treat cancer pain use a stepped approach for cancer pain management. These steps are listed on the following pages. The steps and the recommended relief match the severity of pain a person is having.

STEP 1. MILD PAIN–NONOPIOIDS

The first step to controlling mild pain is through the use of nonopioid drugs. **Nonopioids** are mild pain relievers. They are also called:

- **Analgesics:** examples are acetaminophen or Tylenol
- **Nonsteroidal anti-inflammatory drugs (NSAIDs):** examples are aspirin and ibuprofen (Motrin or Advil). Check with the doctor before using these medicines. NSAIDs can slow bloodclotting, especially if the person with cancer is on chemotherapy.
- **Adjuvants:** examples are antidepressants such as Elavil; anticonvulsants such as Tegretol or Dilantin; and corticosteroids such as dexamethasone and prednisone. These medicines are used to help

enhance the effects of the analgesics, treat symptoms that may increase the pain, and provide pain relief for certain types of pain.

STEP 2. MODERATE PAIN—OPIOIDS

Opioids are drugs that are more potent than nonopioids and more effective for stronger pain. These are also known as narcotics.

If Step 1 drugs do not work, or if the pain is rated as moderate pain, this step deals with what medicines to use. Opioids are often prescribed to be taken with a nonopioid medicine such as those listed in Step 1. Examples of opioids used in this category are codeine, Lortabs, or Percocet.

STEP 3. SEVERE PAIN—OPIOIDS

If the person with cancer is having severe pain, stronger medicines may be needed. A strong opioid can be short acting or long acting. Morphine and Dilaudid are two examples of strong opioids whose effects last three to four hours.

Many pain medicines are also available in "sustained release" (longer-acting) forms that last for eight or twelve hours, such as MS Contin or Oramorph. Kadian is a slow-release pill that lasts for up to 24 hours, and Duragesic is available as a patch that delivers the drug through the skin continuously for 72 hours.

When a patient cannot ingest tablets or liquid because of difficulty swallowing, some medications are taken by putting them inside the cheek or between the cheek and gums. The medicine is absorbed through the lining of the mouth. This is called "transmucosal administration."

Your goals are to:

- call for professional help when it is needed
- understand the medication plan
- make the best use of pain medicines
- ask about changing pain prescriptions as needed
- manage side effects of pain medicines
- do things on your own to prevent and control pain

When to Get Professional Help

Signs and symptoms listed below indicate pain is out of control. Call the doctor or nurse immediately if any of the following conditions exist:

- **Unable to get up or walk because of pain.** A tumor can press on a nerve and cause severe pain, especially when the person moves. Swelling or inflammation around a tumor can push on tender tissues or nerves. In these examples, persons with cancer feel severe pain, may cry out, and may not be able to get up from bed or walk without help.

- **Unable to sleep because of pain.** Poor sleep due to discomfort, aches, and pains is a sure sign that something needs to be done to increase comfort.

- **Crying and upset about feeling pain.** Look for physical responses to pain: tears, closed eyes, knitted eyebrows, wrinkled forehead, grimaced face, clenched fists, or a stiffened chest and back, which is held rigidly and moved slowly. When this happens, or when the person complains about severe pain, call the doctor or nurse immediately.

- **Unwilling to move or muscles are very tense when moving.** Even if he or she does not complain and tries to act as if nothing is wrong, watch how easily he or she moves. People in pain move with great difficulty. Urge the person with cancer to try not to move and not do normal everyday things like getting dressed or getting out of bed.

- **A bone sticks out in an unusual way.** Bones can break or fracture more easily as a person gets older. Cancer that has spread to the bone also increases the risk of a fracture. If a bone sticks out in a new way, report this, even if pain does not immediately follow this event.

- **Decreased appetite because of pain.** Watch for a sudden decrease in appetite. Although appetite is changed by many other factors, do not rule out aches and pains as the cause.

- **Pain continues to be a problem between doses of long-acting medicines** (when six to twelve hours of relief are expected). This is known as "breakthrough pain." Breakthrough pain occurs in between the scheduled times for giving pain medicine.

Know the following facts before you call about an emergency because of severe pain:

- How long has the pain been a problem?___________________
- Where is it located? Is it in more than one area?_____________
- How severe is the pain? Ask the person to use a number from 0 to 10 to describe or rate the pain, where 0 = none, 5 = moderate, and 10 = worst ever. ______________________________
- Is the pain sharp and stabbing or dull and aching? _________
- Does the pain burn or feel like an electric shock? ___________
- Is there any numbness or tingling?_______________________
- How much has this pain interfered with doing normal activities? ____
- Describe any medicines used for pain:
  - Name of medicine(s) ___________________________
  - How much time between doses? ____________________
  - How many pills are to be taken at one time? __________
  - How many doses were taken in the last two days? ________
  - How long do they take to work? ____________________
  - How much relief do they give? _____________________
  - How long does this relief last? _____________________
- What other medicines have been taken or what else has been done to relieve the pain? What were the results? __________ ____

Use the chart on the following page when calling about an emergency because of severe pain (see Table 2 on the next page).

Here's an example of what you might say when calling:

"My brother complains that his pain is getting worse. This morning he refused to get out of bed because his leg hurt so badly at the hip, and it hurts even if he tries to move just a little in bed. He said his pain is an "8" and is sharp. At 6:00 A.M. he took two Percocets but didn't feel any better. The next time for his medicine isn't until noon. We tried a hot water bottle, but it didn't help."

Table 2. Emergency Pain Chart

How long has the pain lasted?	
Where is the pain located? List all areas.	
Rate the severity of the pain. 0 = None, 5 = Moderate, 10 = Worst ever	
Describe the pain: stabbing, dull, aching, burning, and/or like an electric shock.	
Is there numbness or tingling?	
How much has the pain interfered with doing normal activities?	
List:	
Names of medicines	
Times between doses	
How many pills can be taken at one time	
Number of doses taken in last two days	
How long they take to work	
How much relief they give	
How long the relief lasts	
List other medicines taken or other things done to relieve the pain and how much they helped.	

When to get immediate help for effects of pain medicines

A drug reaction is a different type of emergency related to pain control. If the person with cancer is allergic to pain medicines, or the pain medicines are too strong, professional help is needed.

Call the doctor or nurse immediately if any of the following symptoms occur when taking pain medicines:

- **Hallucinations (hearing or seeing things that are not there).**
- **Ringing or buzzing in the ears.**
- **Confusion or being "out of it."**
- **Difficulty waking up even when others try to wake the person.**
- **Severe trembling, uncontrolled muscle movements, or convulsions (seizures).**
- **Unable to hold urine or stool when this was not a problem in the past.**
- **Unable to urinate despite feeling the need to urinate.**
- **Nausea or vomiting with no relief.**
- **Hives, itching, skin rash, or swelling of the face.**
- **Feeling anxious or "fidgety."**
- **Slow breathing (less than eight breaths per minute) or very shallow breathing (short breaths that don't take in much air).**

Know the following facts before you call about an emergency caused by pain medicines:

- What pain medicine was taken over the last few days? ________
  ____
- How much medicine was taken?__________________________
- How often was it taken? ___________________________

Most of the symptoms on the "call now" list indicate a drug reaction is causing a problem with the central nervous system, the gastrointestinal tract, the urinary tract, or the skin, and the body's normal functioning is severely impaired. Either the medicine is too strong or there is an uncommon allergic reaction.

Side effects like those on the list demand immediate action. When you call and report these symptoms, the doctor or nurse will most likely want to see the person with cancer right away, or they will send emergency help to you. After evaluating what is happening, they can give medicines to clear any drugs out of the body. They can also prescribe other ways to calm the central nervous system and reverse an allergic reaction.

Problems with drug reactions are not common. When they do happen, it is important to get help right away.

When symptoms are not an emergency, but should be reported

Some symptoms are not considered an emergency but should still be reported during regular office hours. Call the doctor or nurse if any of the following conditions exist:

No relief after taking pain medicine three times, as prescribed. Call and discuss the pain problem with the doctor or nurse.

Some pain relief, but there is still significant pain after one or two days. The physician or nurse needs to reevaluate the amount or type of pain medicine prescribed.

A new type of pain, pain in new locations, or new pain when moving or sitting. Report pain in new locations. New pains may need to be evaluated before the next regularly scheduled clinic visit.

Numbness, tingling, or burning sensations that are new. They can signal an early problem with the nervous system or with the amount of medicine being taken. Report these so the doctor or nurse can locate the cause and make the necessary changes in the treatment plan. These types of pain may need to be treated with medicines other than commonly prescribed drugs and analgesics. When a tumor invades nerves, it might cause a feeling of numbness, tingling, burning, or a short electrical shock. Low doses of antidepressants often help relieve these symptoms, help sleep, and even readjust chemicals in the spinal cord, which help control pain.

Medicines for breakthrough pain are used three to four times a day in addition to the regular pain medicines. When breakthrough pain occurs, the doctor may change the medicine schedule, may prescribe extra doses to be given "as needed," or may prescribe a different type of pain medicine in addition to the regular pain medicine.

Tremors or involuntary jerking motions while awake or asleep. These motions can indicate a need for the doctor to adjust the pain medication.

What You Can Do to Help

If you decide a pain problem is not an emergency and that a drug reaction has not occurred, there are several things you can do to help manage cancer pain:

- make the best use of pain medicines
- understand the medication plan
- ask about changing pain prescriptions as needed
- manage common side effects of pain medicine
- do things to prevent or control pain on your own

Make the best use of medicines

If the person needs medicine on a regular basis, be sure you are using the pain medicine correctly and controlling pain before it becomes severe.

Give the pain medicine at regular times, as prescribed by the doctor. When pain occurs regularly and not just once or twice a day, give the pain medicine on a consistent schedule to keep enough medicine in the bloodstream to keep the pain away. Encourage the person with cancer not to wait too long to take it.

For example, suppose the pain medicine is prescribed "every four to six hours as needed." You can give pain medicine anytime after four hours. However, do not wait longer than six hours because the pain may become so bad the prescribed amount will not give full relief.

Give the pain medicine before the pain builds up. When pain occurs regularly and not just once or twice a day, pain control is more difficult. It also takes longer to achieve control if pain is allowed to build to a severe level. Give the pain medicine on a regular basis. People need to take pain medicine to avoid a pain crisis, just like diabetics need to take insulin to avoid a "sugar" crisis.

Taking medicine with the same hours between doses prevents "peaks and valleys" and keeps a steady supply of medicine in the body. You may even find you can decrease the amount of pain medicine because the person with pain is more confident that pain can be controlled.

Continue to give the pain medicine during the night. Try not to go longer than eight to ten hours without giving medicine during the night, unless the person is taking "sustained release" (longer-acting) preparation medicines such as MS Contin, Oxycontin, or Duragesic. Too much time between doses means the amount of medicine in the body keeps dropping and the level of pain increases. The person with cancer will then need more of the medicine so it will return to the right level. Giving a dose of pain medicine in the middle of the night helps you prevent breakthrough pain.

Do not stop the pain medicine suddenly if it has been taken for a number of weeks. In a few people with cancer, if pain medicine is stopped suddenly, the body may experience a strong reaction. It expects a steady flow of these medicines into the bloodstream. Symptoms can occur in the same way as when one suddenly stops smoking cigarettes or drinking coffee. Symptoms, such as shakiness, nausea, sweating, or headache, are less likely to occur if the pain medicine is stopped slowly over a few days and under the direction of a physician. Increasing the length of time between doses and taking lower doses of the pain medicine lets the body be weaned away from the medicines in a gentle manner.

Doing these things also helps relieve other problems that can increase pain, such as muscle tension, lack of sleep, and emotional distress.

Ask the doctor or nurse the following questions:

- What if the medicine wears off and pain returns, but it is too early for the next dose of pain medicine? ________________

- Can more medicine be taken in addition to the prescribed amount if the pain is not relieved, or must we first call the doctor?

  ____

- What can I do if pain wakes him or her up during the night? __

  ____

- What should I do if a dose is accidentally skipped? __________

  ____

- Is this a medicine that we can crush or have the pharmacist mix in a liquid so it's easier to swallow? (Some longer-acting medicines, such as MS Contin, should not be crushed because all the medicine will be absorbed at one time. This could be dangerous when the purpose of the medicine is to be delivered in a time-released fashion.) ____

Understand the medication plan

Understanding how and when the doctor and nurse want you to give pain medicines is the key to successful pain control and prevention. There are three different pain control plans, and you can ask which one you are on.

PLAN 1: TAKE MEDICINE AS NEEDED (GIVE PRN)

Pain medicines can be ordered "as needed," which is sometimes written as "give prn." For example, the bottle may be labeled "take every three to four hours as needed" or "take every six hours as needed." This means the person with pain can decide when to take the medicine but should not take it more than the lowest number of hours listed on the instruction label (see *Appendix* on page 270). If he or she needs the medicine before this lowest number, discuss the problem with a doctor or nurse.

For example, if the prescription is to "take every three to four hours as needed," the person with pain can take the medicine every three hours and do so consistently, especially if the pain starts to come back three hours after the last dose. They can also wait four hours or longer if pain does not return. Writing down the times the person with pain takes pain medicine helps the doctor or nurse understand what is happening and adjust the prescription and timing to achieve maximum pain relief.

Taking medicine "as needed" also means the person can take a dose and then wait to take another one until they feel the first inkling of pain or before they begin an activity that stimulates the pain problem. Some people learn exactly what brings on their pain, such as bending over the stove while cooking or bending over the dryer while doing laundry.

PLAN 2: TAKE MEDICINE WITH EQUAL NUMBER OF HOURS BETWEEN DOSES

Know when to give a medicine ordered for a certain number of times per day, such as two, four, or six times a day. If the medicine is ordered for a certain number of times per day (not for a certain number of hours), then start with the time the person wakes up and divide the 24-hour day into equal spaces. For example, if a medicine is ordered as "take twice a day" and the person is usually awake at 9:00 A.M. then give a dose at 9:00 A.M. and again at 9:00 P.M. The times do not have to be exact, but try to divide the day into even sections. Some examples of dividing the 24-hour day if the person awakens at 9:00 A.M. are shown in Table 3 on the next page.

Table 3. Medication Schedule

Dose Ordered Four times a day	Dose Ordered Six times a day
9:00 A.M.	9:00 A.M.
3:00 P.M.	1:00 P.M.
9:00 P.M.	5:00 P.M.
3:00 A.M.	9:00 P.M.
	1:00 A.M.
	5:00 A.M.

PLAN 3: TAKE EXTRA MEDICINE WHEN PAIN BREAKS THROUGH BEFORE THE NEXT MEDICINE IS DUE

Treat breakthrough pain to prevent its return. Usually, there is a separate prescription just for when this happens, or the doctor may advise the person with pain to take an analgesic medicine (the first step in the stepped approach) if pain comes back too soon but it is not time to take the strongest pain medicine itself (see pages 136–137).

If breakthrough pain happens for the first time, make sure the person is taking pain medicines as frequently as ordered. Sometimes taking the pain medicine more consistently (the same number of hours between doses) and more frequently (for example, if ordered every four to six hours, then take every four hours) around the clock prevents breakthrough pain.

Ask the doctor about changing pain prescriptions, times, and doses

If the person with cancer is taking the medicine as prescribed and is still feeling significant pain or is really bothered by the side effects from the pain medicine, ask the doctor if there are other pain medicines or ways to take them that might help more.

Ask about increasing the amount of medicine. Sometimes there is just too little medicine in the body to prevent pain. If so, the doctor may increase the pain medicine until the right amount is discovered.

Ask about shortening the time between doses of pain medicine. Perhaps the right amount of pain medicine is not kept in the bloodstream because the pain medicine isn't taken often enough. If so, the doctor may shorten the time between doses to increase the level of the medicine in the body. Talk to the doctor before shortening time between doses. Be sure to indicate what time the pain medicine was taken and at what time after (how many hours) the pain returned.

Ask about taking short-acting or immediate-release opioids for breakthrough pain. Faster-acting pain medicines can be ordered to stop breakthrough pain. The long-acting dose of pain medicine can be increased if the breakthrough pain occurs more than twice. Sometimes people need to have their dose almost doubled to prevent breakthrough pain from happening again.

Ask about giving the same medicine in a different form or about using a different technique to give the medicine. An example is giving medicine through an IV line that you can take care of at home.

There are many new ways to take pain medicines. Here are some of the different ways pain medicine can be given:

- *Liquid pain medicine:* If someone with pain cannot eat solid foods, he or she may have trouble swallowing pills. Some pain medicines are available in liquid form. A pharmacist can also mix a liquid syrup with one or more pain medicines in it, which can be given with a measuring spoon.
- *Skin patches:* A recent advance is the "transdermal" skin patch, which is placed on the body (chest or back) and delivers a medicine through the skin for up to 72 hours. You change the patch every 72 hours.
- *Time release pills:* There are also pills that give pain relief for a long time, such as 12- or 24-hour, time-released tablets of morphine.
- *Rectal suppositories:* Pain medicine also comes in rectal suppositories—or can be prepared in suppository form by the pharmacist. Once placed in the body, they melt and are absorbed into the body. They are helpful to people who cannot swallow pills.

- *Single injections into muscles:* Pain medicine can be received by injection into the muscle. If the idea of a needle scares the person with pain, a thinner or smaller needle may be used. Many family caregivers learn to give injections to family members or friends.
- *Subcutaneous (SubQ) needles attached under the skin:* A small needle can be placed just under the skin by a health care worker. Medicine is given through this line every few hours by a family caregiver. These lines can also be hooked to pumps, which deliver the medicine at regular times. The needle has to be changed and reinserted at a new site every few days by a nurse.
- *IV lines inserted into large veins:* These are called Hickmans, Broviacs, or peripherally inserted central catheters (PICCs). These are all placed into large arm veins. The tubing comes outside of the skin a few inches, and medicine is given much like with an IV line. The dressings are changed by nurses at the clinic or at home.
- *Implanted ports under the skin:* An implanted port such as Mediport is a new way to get medicine into a large vein in the chest. These ports are about one inch wide and one inch deep, circular, and made of metal. They are usually surgically placed under the skin of the upper chest, and a nurse can find its exact placement by gently pushing on the skin and feeling the small round disc. The nurse cleans the skin with a solution and injects medicine into the port, which flows into the vein. Sometimes the site can be used to draw blood for laboratory tests.
- *IV-infusing pumps attached to implanted ports:* There are also small, portable pumps with IV lines that can be carried on a belt. They are run on batteries and can deliver the medicine evenly day and night. Home health nurses or home IV nurses can manage this and teach family caregivers how to care for the pump and line. Some people with cancer give themselves medicine through these lines as well.
- *Epidural catheters near the spine:* Anesthesiologists can put epidural catheters near the spine to deliver medicines, and family caregivers can be taught how to give medicines through these catheters or a pump may be used to give the medicine continuously.

Ask about adding other medicines or treatments

The doctor may combine several types of pain medicine that work in different ways to give relief.

- *Changing pain medicines.* If pain persists after trying the above suggestions, it is time for the person with cancer, caregiver, and health care staff to discuss another pain medication plan.
- *The use of radiation therapy for pain.* Sometimes radiation is prescribed to shrink a tumor that is causing pain. Treatments usually are given daily, lasting from a few days up to four or five weeks to help control pain caused by a tumor.
- *A referral to a pain clinic to be seen by specialists in pain management.* Universities and large hospitals have special clinics to evaluate and treat chronic pain. Most pain clinics require a doctor refer the person with pain to them.

  Doctors, nurses, counselors, and pharmacists at a pain clinic know a lot about special procedures for managing pain. For example, an anesthesiologist can give a nerve block that stops a feeling of pain for a short time until other methods are prescribed, or the nerve block can be given to last a long time. Another advantage of a pain clinic is the staff there might prescribe a combination of two or three medicines that relieve different types of pain. If there is no pain clinic at your local hospital, you can ask for a referral to a pain clinic at another hospital. You can also call the pain clinic at another hospital and ask how referrals are handled.

Manage the more common side effects of pain medicine

Not all people react the same way to pain medicines. However, certain side effects are very common. Watch for these and deal with them early.

Prevent constipation with diet, liquids, stool softeners, and laxatives. Opioid pain medicines cause constipation by slowing down the bowel, which leads to loss of water from the stool. This makes the stool hard and difficult to pass. Stool softeners and laxatives can help put water back into the stool, making it less hard and easier to pass. When opioid medicines are taken, the person is usually placed on a bowel program to prevent constipation. Ask your doctor or nurse about a bowel program.

Try a product such as Milk of Magnesia if stool softeners and laxatives do not work and the person with cancer has not had a bowel movement in two to three days. You may have to increase the number of stool softeners and stimulants taken every day or give a mild enema. See the chapter *Constipation* (pages 165–173), which describes different ways to prevent constipation.

Serve food with high fiber content, such as prunes, fresh fruit and vegetables, or bran. These add bulk to what is inside the intestines and attract water back into the intestines, which softens the stool. Also, offer fluids—as much as eight to ten glasses a day.

Avoid foods that tend to cause constipation, such as cheese or chocolate.

Relieve a dry mouth with crushed ice, hard candy, and frequent rinses with water or products that do not contain alcohol.

Relieve painful dry nasal passages by humidifying the air or breathing in warm moisture from a sink full of warm water. Saline drops or Ocean Nasal Spray can be purchased at a pharmacy and are helpful.

Avoid an upset stomach by taking medicine with food, unless instructed to do otherwise by the pharmacist.

Relieve mild itching by gently rubbing with a cool cloth. Mild itching for a few days may occur. If the itching persists beyond few days or becomes severe, call the doctor or nurse.

Expect drowsiness for a few days when pain medicine is started or increased. If sleepiness increases just after starting or increasing pain medicine, wait about three days. Sometimes sleepiness happens because a person is finally getting pain relief and needs to catch up on missed rest, or the body needs time to adjust to new medicines or doses. If sleepiness is a concern, offer beverages with caffeine in them, if allowed. Discourage driving a car or operating power tools since opioids slow the responses—just as alcohol does. If the drowsiness lasts longer than a week, contact the doctor so it can be evaluated and corrected. If drowsiness is extreme and you cannot awaken the person, call the doctor or nurse immediately.

Prevent and control pain on your own

There are many things you can do on your own to help prevent and control pain.

MANAGING PAIN MEDICINE

Set an alarm as a reminder to administer pain medicine. This reminds you to give the pain medicine or reminds the person with cancer to take the medicine.

Use a medicine tray or pill box with slots for time of day to hold the medicines. These are plastic boxes with squares for each day of the week and slots for dose times. Many people fill the box for the whole week. You can also use an egg carton and mark each slot with the name of the day of the week and the time the pain medicine is to be given that day.

Telephone the pharmacy before going to fill the pain prescription. Some pharmacies do not carry all pain medicines. They may have to special order it or send you to another store.

Use the same pharmacy, if possible. If you use the same pharmacists, they will understand what the medication plan is, how it is working, and have suggestions on how to handle side effects. They will also know what pain medicines to keep on hand and can answer many of your questions about the medicines. They will also be able to warn you about possible "drug interactions." Drug interactions occur when one drug affects how another drug works.

Keep at least a five-day supply of pain medicine. Call the doctor for a new prescription before the last pain medicine is given. If you are planning to be out of town, be certain to have a sufficient supply until your planned return.

HELPING TO CONTROL PAIN

Use warm showers, baths, hot water bottles, or warm washcloths. Heat relaxes the muscles and gives a sense of comfort. Do not set heating pads on high because they can burn the skin. Do not place them over or near areas where radiation marks are on the skin, even when radiation treatments are finished. If the person with cancer is wearing a patch that provides pain medicine, ask the doctor before using heat since heat can increase the amount of drug released from the patch.

Use cool cloths or ice. Cooling the skin and muscles can soothe pain, especially pain that comes from inflammation or swelling. For example, many people like using a cool washcloth on their foreheads when they have a headache.

Position the person carefully with pillows and soft seat cushions.

Massage sore spots, such as the neck and shoulders.

Encourage the person to avoid lifting or straining.

Encourage him or her to use deep breathing exercises. Breathing deeply, slowly, and quietly helps the mind and body to relax, which helps decrease pain. Use tape recordings or follow instructions in books on relaxation. Ask the health care team about these techniques, or read the chapter *Anxiety* (pages 88–99) to learn more about relaxation.

Encourage pleasant, involving activities. This helps to take the mind off of the pain. Different people are distracted by different activities. One person may be distracted by watching television or going through a catalog. Another may be distracted by listening to music or visiting with friends.

Ask for help with tasks. Now is the time for both you and the person with cancer not to overdo it. Get others to lend a hand. Do not be shy about asking for help! It is part of your job as a caregiver to get help when you need it.

Encourage doing activities when he or she feels most comfortable. Plan activities during times when the person with pain is feeling best and is most awake.

Keep a diary, rate the pain, and keep notes on what makes it worse or better. Writing down what makes the pain worse or better helps you and the person with cancer plan how to manage this problem. Keep track of the times, amounts, and names of pain medicines given and use words such as ache, pressure, burning, dull, and sharp to describe the pain. If you bring this diary with you to doctor appointments, it helps the staff understand what you are doing, and helps them make recommendations about treatments.

Avoid stressful events when possible. Emotional stress and anxiety increases awareness and sensitivity to pain. If you can cancel certain events that are stressful, do so. See the chapters on anxiety and depression for ways to control emotional stress.

Encourage attending a support group meeting for people with cancer or educational session in your area. Many people with cancer enjoy these, and family and friends are welcome. To find out where and when local support groups meet, ask your local American Cancer Society office or look in the telephone book. You can also ask nurses, doctors, or social workers at your local hospital about support groups in your area.

Possible Obstacles

Here are some common obstacles that have stopped others from giving (or taking) pain medicines:

"I'm afraid of addiction."

People who take opioids for cancer pain do not become addicted. In fact, if their pain is treated effectively, it decreases the risk of addiction.

People who are "addicts" take drugs for a "high" or an altered state of mind. People who take opioids for cancer pain take them to get relief from physical pain. People who are not addicts before they take opioids for cancer pain do not become addicts later. Remember the medicine is being used for pain control and not for a psychological "high."

Even if you understand your friend or family member is not addicted, others may not. Tell them this medicine is part of the medical treatment and absolutely crucial to the person's quality of life and ability to do what is most important to them.

"I want to 'save' the pain medicine and give it when the pain is severe."

Taking pain medicine for mild discomfort now does not affect how well it will work in the future or when the pain gets worse.

Don't hold back the pain medicines you take today in order to save up if more pain medicine is needed later. In fact, it takes more medicine to treat the pain that is uncontrolled than it does to prevent pain from building up.

People sometimes need to increase their doses of pain medicine. Their need for more medicine does not mean they are becoming "immune" to pain medicines, or they need more and more medicine to control the same level of pain. These people need more medication because the pain has changed. Actually, there is no real dose limit for most of the pain drugs a person can take. A few do have upper limits. If the person with pain reaches that limit, the doctor can change to a different pain medicine. The doctor knows when it is right to change a medicine.

If pain is controlled now, you and the person with pain can be less worried about controlling it later because you know the medicines do work. Also, taking enough medicine now helps the person with pain relax and preserve his or her strength.

"No one wants to hear about my pain."

Family and friends may seem uninterested because they feel helpless. Doctors and nurses who specialize in pain, such as those in a pain clinic or hospice, do understand pain problems. Talk to them if you are feeling alone with these problems.

"He doesn't want to take any morphine because he thinks that means he's dying. Only people who are close to death take morphine."

Morphine is not reserved for the dying. It is an effective medicine for many types of cancer pain. Taking it does not mean a person is near death. It is also used to control chronic pain during earlier phases of the disease. Some people go back to work and do their regular daily activities because the morphine is so effective. It lets them return to pain-free lives.

Think of other obstacles that could interfere with carrying out your plan

What additional roadblocks could get in the way of doing the things recommended in this chapter? For example, will the person with cancer cooperate? Will other people help? How will you explain your needs to other people? Do you have the time and energy to carry out the plan?

Develop plans for getting around these roadblocks using the six problem-solving steps discussed in the first section of this book (see pages xi–xvi).

Carrying Out and Adjusting Your Plan

Checking on results

Keep track of the pain level. You can do this by asking the person you are caring for to tell you how severe the pain is. Use the same terms each time you do this so you can compare one time with another. This helps you evaluate how effective the pain control program is and to notice changes. For example, you might want to use the words "worst ever," "severe," "bad," "moderate," "mild," and "none at all" each time. The person who is telling you about the pain can choose which word fits best or even say it is between the words (for example, "It is between severe and bad."). Another way to do this is to think of a 10-inch ruler, where 10 is the worst pain ever, 0 is no pain, and 5 is moderate pain. The person can give you a number to fit his or her pain. You can use the chart on page 157 (Table 4) to help keep track of the level of pain.

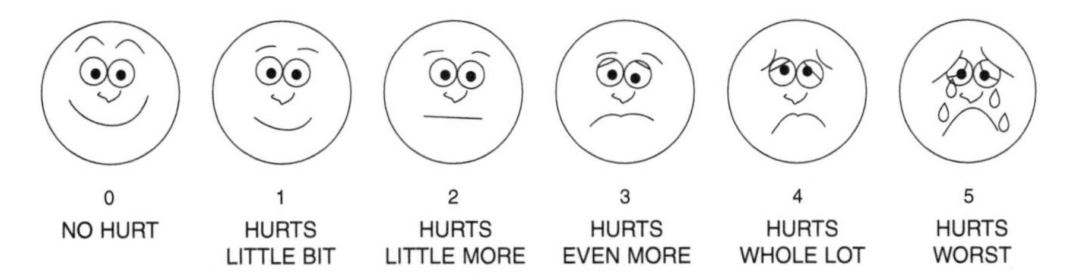

Wong-Baker FACES Pain Rating Scale. (From Wong DL, Hockenberry-Eaton M, Wilson D, Winkelstein ML, Schwartz P: *Wong's Essentials of Pediatric Nursing, 6/e,* St. Louis, 2001, P. 1301. Copyrighted by Mosby, Inc. Reprinted by permission.)

If these ratings are to be meaningful, it is essential the person with pain understand you fully accept his or her ratings. Pain can be judged only by the person who has it. The person with cancer has to feel you trust and accept what is said about pain—or he or she won't cooperate, or will give incorrect information.

If your plan doesn't work...

If problems with pain are getting worse, review the *When to Get Professional Help* section of this chapter (pages 138–142). If you decide to call the doctor or nurse, tell them what was done to deal with pain and discuss what else could be done.

If you do not think you need to talk with a doctor or nurse immediately or during regular office hours about pain, then ask yourself if you are doing everything you can to make the best use of medicines and to control pain on your own. Review this chapter to be sure you are doing everything you can to deal with this problem.

Remember: Cancer pain can be very well controlled. Do not accept anything less than the best pain control.

If you feel the medical staff is not listening to your concerns or is not able to give adequate pain control, you can ask them to refer you to a cancer pain specialist. These are physicians who specialize in cancer pain and can usually be found at cancer centers, or they may be local physicians who are involved in hospice care.

Table 4. Pain Record

Time of Day	Pain Rating (Rate 0-10)	What was the person doing when pain was triggered (e.g., walking, exercising, sleeping)	Medication taken and dose	What other things were done to relieve pain (e.g., heat, meditation, etc.)	Pain Rating after treatment (Rate 0-10)	How long it took to get relief
Midnight						
1:00 A.M.						
2:00						
3:00						
4:00						
5:00						
6:00						
7:00						
8:00						
9:00						
10:00						
11:00						
Noon						
1:00 P.M.						
2:00						
3:00						
4:00						
5:00						
6:00						
7:00						
8:00						
9:00						
10:00						
11:00						

Pain Scale: 0 = none; 5 = moderate; 10 = worst ever

Confusion and Seizures

Understanding the Condition

Mental confusion during cancer treatments is not common, but if it does happen, it is upsetting to both the person with cancer and caregivers. It can also cause communication problems that are frustrating to both. Sometimes, this even leads the person with cancer to stop trying to communicate. Family caregivers may be tempted to give up as well, but they should understand steps can be taken to cope with these problems.

Mental confusion and communication problems can be caused by medicines, strokes, changes in body chemistry, or the presence of cancer in the brain. In addition, lack of sleep or adequate rest can add to a person's disorientation (not knowing where one is or who other people are), as can new and unfamiliar surroundings.

Although very rare, seizures are another possible problem with brain functioning in the people with cancer. When a seizure does occur, both caregivers and people with cancer can become very frightened. So, preparing in advance is wise, especially if the treatment staff warns that a seizure may happen.

Your goals are to:

- call for professional help if needed
- help the person with cancer avoid becoming confused
- make it as easy as possible for the person to understand both you and others
- know what to do if a seizure occurs

When to Get Professional Help

Call the doctor or nurse if any of the following conditions exist:

- **A sudden change in ability to speak after a new medicine is started.** This should be reported to a physician or nurse. The medicine may be the cause of the problem, and the doctor may need to adjust the doses and the medicines being taken.
- **Mental confusion that is new or increased.**
- **Any change such as clouded thinking or not knowing where they are.**
- **A sudden, dramatic change in personality.**
- **If someone is outgoing one week but very quiet the next, or vice versa.** The cause may be a physical change in the brain, emotional problems such as depression, a medicine being taking, or a stroke.
- **A sudden change in ability to care for himself or herself.**
- **If the person with cancer suddenly needs help to manage routine tasks.** Tasks, such as dressing or washing, which used to be managed alone, may indicate a need for a doctor's evaluation. Call the physician's office and ask for an evaluation to see if there is a physical cause.
- **Falling because of confusion.** Mental confusion increases the likelihood people will not know where they are. Climbing out of bed or getting up and walking can cause a fall. Ask a nurse to come to the house and help you make the rooms safer. If the person does fall, make him or her comfortable on the floor using pillows and blankets and then call for help. For example, the staff at a local fire company can come out and gently lift the person back into bed; they have the strength and they know how to move people safely.
- **A change in ability to talk, such as long pauses or slurred words while speaking.** Changes in the ability to speak can happen suddenly or over a short period of time, such as several days. Problems with speaking can result from a stroke in which parts of the brain do not get enough blood or oxygen. Recognizing

changes in speech may be difficult because he or she may be sleeping more and talking less. Even so, watch for changes such as a person who uses complete sentences suddenly speaking in short words, using sentences that make no sense, or babbling. Other symptoms of a stroke are numbness on one side of the face or body; inability to move one side of the face when smiling, frowning, or speaking; and inability to move a hand, arm, or leg.

Have the answers to the following questions ready when you call the doctor or nurse:

- When did the confusion or word slurring start? ____________
  ____
- Were any new medicines started? If so, which ones, when, and at what dosage?____________________________
- Has the person changed where he or she is living? __________
  ____
- Have other changes occurred in person's setting? If so, what are they? ____________________________

Here is an example of what someone might say when calling for professional help:

"My mother is Dr. Lindquist's patient. This morning she suddenly started slurring her words and wasn't sure where she was."

What You Can Do to Help

Here are three things you can do to deal with confusion and communication problems:

1. Make it as easy as possible for the person to understand you and others.
2. Help the person avoid becoming confused.
3. Know what to do if a seizure occurs.

Make it as easy as possible for the person to understand both you and others.

Use simple words and short sentences. Short words and sentences are easy to understand. Also, ask questions one at a time, and wait for an answer. Try not to give complex choices, either. Do not ask questions such as "Do you want to lie down now or have Fred visit?" Instead, just ask "Do you want Fred to visit now?" However, avoid treating the adult like a child or using baby talk.

Use a picture or the "real thing" to get your message across. If the person does not seem to understand a simple question, show something to help get the message across. For example, if you want to know if he or she would like something to drink, show a glass of liquid.

Keep other noise down in the room. If others are talking and a TV or radio is blaring, it will be hard for anyone to hear a conversation or a question. Keep this in mind if the person is having difficulty understanding someone else's speech.

Explain to visitors or other caregivers how they can help the person with cancer hear and understand better. Explain that hearing or talking is a problem, and show what you do to cope with any confusion and to improve communication.

Explain what is happening before you turn, move, or help the confused person. It helps a confused person to know what is going to happen before a change such as getting out of bed or serving a meal. However, try not to treat the person like a child. Just use simple words and explain what is going to happen.

Try not to argue. It is easy to lose patience with someone who is not mentally clear or keeps forgetting what you say. However, arguing can increase anxiety and actually make it harder for him or her to understand what you are saying.

Help the person avoid becoming confused.

Try to keep the person awake during the day and asleep during the night. Many people who are very sick get night and day mixed up, and this can add to their confusion. Try to keep the person awake during the day so he or she can sleep during the night. This way, certain routines, such as mealtime or bath time, will not seem so disorienting.

Use a night-light in the room to help the person see and remember where he or she is. A person who is a little confused can sometimes wake up and not remember where he or she is. A night-light gives just enough illumination to help the person see and get oriented.

Keep the person's surroundings as familiar as possible. Unfamiliar surroundings or people may cause confusion. If the confused person goes to a nursing home or a hospital, take pictures, photographs, favorite pillows, or covers into the new setting to retain some familiarity.

Keep a clock and a calendar within sight. It is easy to lose track of the time of day and the day of the week. Clocks and calendars help to remind all of us about the time.

Continue giving medicines on a regular schedule. Some medicines may be prescribed to reduce confusion. One example is steroids, such as prednisone, which decrease swelling or inflammation in the brain. If confusion or problems with talking are caused by a cancer in the brain, it is important to keep giving medicines that keep any swelling from getting worse.

Ask if medicine doses need to be lowered because of weight loss. Some medicines have different doses for people with different weights. If someone is losing weight, the dose may be too large, which might cause confusion. Perhaps the doses of these drugs could be lowered without losing their desired effects.

Know what to do if a seizure occurs.

Place a soft washcloth in the person's mouth. The purpose of placing something in the mouth is to prevent the person from biting his or her tongue or lips while the seizure lasts.

Avoid putting your hands in the person's mouth. Do not try holding the person's tongue or mouth with your hands. Most likely, you will be bitten. Instead, place the soft washcloth inside the person's mouth when it opens.

Put pillows on both sides of the body. Pillows will help keep the person in place and help prevent falling out of bed.

Pad any side rails on the bed with soft blankets. Metal side rails on hospital beds can hurt and bruise a person when he or she bumps into them. Padding the side rails is a good idea if you expect a problem with seizures.

Turn lights down to soft lighting. Soft illumination is calming, and people usually rest better when they are not squinting into bright lights.

Tell others how to handle seizures. Keep a list near the person's bed of what to do if a seizure occurs. Keep a soft washcloth nearby. If volunteers or others who are not the usual caregivers stay with the person, they can read this list and know what to do.

Possible Obstacles

Here are some common obstacles that other caregivers have faced:

"Why bother to explain anything? He doesn't know where he is or who I am."

Confusion can come and go, so you will not always know if the person is confused at that particular moment. Explain things, and talk with him as an adult.

"Why talk about the past? She can't even remember where she is now."

Remembering the past might be easier for her than remembering what happened yesterday. In general, this is true for many older adults (those older than 85 years old). Talking about the past can be pleasant and comforting as well, and it can bring tears as well as laughter. If other friends or family are present, they also will enjoy the stories and learn more about her.

"I feel so sad that he doesn't know who I am."

It is sad to lose the sense that he knew you before and now he does not. This can make you feel like you have lost someone. Maybe there were things you wanted to say or do together, and you now wonder if it is worth it. Say those things anyway, and hope your words are understood as coming from you (because you cannot always be sure he does not know who you are).

Think of other obstacles that could interfere with carrying out your plan

What additional roadblocks could get in the way of doing the things recommended in this chapter? For example, will the person with cancer cooperate? Will other people help? How will you explain your needs to other people? Do you have the time and energy to carry out the plan?

Develop plans for getting around these roadblocks using the six problem-solving steps discussed in the first section of this book (see pages xi–xvi).

Carrying Out and Adjusting Your Plan

Carrying out your plan

Be patient and creative. It will take time to discover the best ways to communicate with someone whose mental abilities are limited. Also, be realistic in your expectations.

Checking on results

Look for signs the person recognizes you and understands what you have said. Keep track of what causes any such improvement.

If your plan doesn't work...

If communication and confusion remain problems, ask the doctor or nurse for further suggestions and guidance. They have experience communicating with people who are confused and will know what you can realistically hope to achieve.

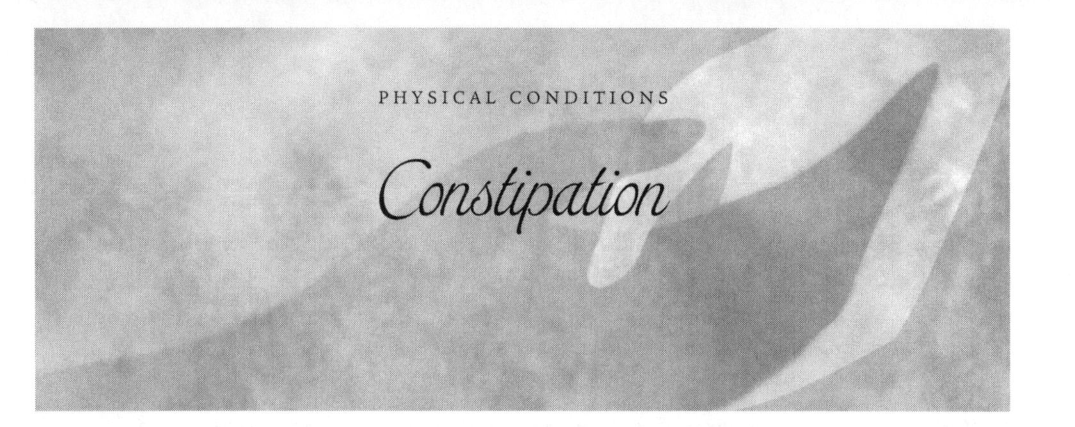

Understanding the Condition

Most constipation can be prevented. This takes planning and regular attention to what is eaten. It may also involve taking preventive medicine–if it is prescribed. Since you are with the person daily, you are key to managing and preventing this uncomfortable symptom. Because this is a sensitive subject for many people, tact and sensitivity is important to get information about the symptoms and to carry out prescribed treatments. You will need to keep in close contact with health professionals to solve this problem.

Constipation occurs when bowel movements happen less often than usual and when stools are hard or difficult to move. Constipation can be caused by medicines used to treat cancer, narcotics (opioids), emotional stress, changes in diet, or decreases in activity. Constipation is a common problem for people who are weak, spend a lot of time in bed, and are not eating. Even if the person with cancer isn't eating much, the body still makes waste, and regular bowel movements are necessary. Constipation can also be very uncomfortable.

When persons with cancer are constipated, they often have decreased appetite or feel bloated and might have abdominal cramps. These feelings add to their discomfort.

Your goals are to:

- call for professional help when it is needed
- help relieve the constipation
- help prevent constipation in the future

When to Get Professional Help

It is important to report constipation symptoms to the doctor or nurse because they could indicate other problems. For example, a tumor could be pressing on a part of the bowel and preventing that part from allowing stool to pass through it in a normal pattern.

Call the doctor or nurse if any of the following conditions exist:

- **The normal routine was once a day and he or she has not had a bowel movement in three or four days** OR **the normal routine was once every other day and he or she has not had a bowel movement in four or five days.** Constipation becomes more uncomfortable as it continues. If it is allowed to continue for more than a few days, it will also be more difficult to reverse.
- **Severe straining on the toilet.**
- **Severe abdominal pain or an abdomen that feels harder than normal and very full** OR **red blood around the outside of the stools or problems with hemorrhoids.** These can all be signs of constipation that needs medical attention.

When you call, it is important to report all the symptoms plus the usual bowel pattern and the day and type of the last movement. This helps the doctor or nurse decide on what medicines could help and advise you on other measures to take to help relieve the problem. For example, if the doctor or nurse knows there are smears of stool on the clothes or the person with cancer feels full in the rectal area, then they know the lower bowel needs to be evacuated and a laxative or stool softener needs to be prescribed to help with the emptying of the lower bowel in the future.

The doctor or nurse may ask you the following questions, which helps them assess whether the constipation is increasing in severity and whether there is stool close to the rectum but the muscles are not moving the stool out.

Know the following facts before you call the doctor or nurse:

- How often are the person's usual bowel movements?_________
- When was the last bowel movement? What did it look like?____
  ____

Reporting what the last bowel movement looked like (watery or dry) tells the health professional if food is being digested properly and if the stool has enough water in it as it passes through the long digestive and intestinal tract. In addition, color is important to report. Very dark stools could indicate blood in the stool.

- Does the person normally take medicines to help move the bowels, such as laxatives, stool softeners, Metamucil, Citrucel, herbals, or suppositories? If yes, what kind and how often? ______________

  ____

- Does feeling constipated interfere with normal activities such as walking or eating? ______________________________________

  The degree to which the constipation is interfering with the person's comfort and activities is important to report because it is an indication of how severe the constipation is and how important it is to treat quickly.

- What other symptoms are there?

  ____distention or bloating of the abdomen

  ____pressure or sense of fullness in the rectal area

  ____small, frequent "smears" of stool

  ____small amounts of loose stools or "leaking"

  ____rectal pain with a bowel movement

  ____constantly feeling the need to have a bowel movement but unable to pass stool

  ____small amounts of loose stool or diarrhea

  ____nausea

Answers to questions about other symptoms help the doctor or nurse understand the condition. If there is no bowel movement for days, but small amounts of diarrhea occur, they may recommend a gentle enema or a visit to the clinic for a rectal exam and further assessment.

- What medications were taken in the last two or three days?______

  ____

  Be sure to mention any medicines that are being taken, especially:

  · narcotics (opioids or pain pills)

  · laxatives

  · chemotherapy

  Some medicines can interrupt normal bowel activity, and the doctor or nurse will recognize which drugs could be contributing to constipation.

- How much food and liquid was consumed during the last 24 hours?

  ____

  If doctor or nurse knows about food and fluid intake, they can judge if the constipation is an emergency requiring a clinic visit. If they decide the constipation is not an emergency, they may suggest an increase in fluids as well as many of the actions that are listed on the following pages.

Here is an example of what you might say when calling:

"My mother hasn't had a bowel movement for four days. She feels like she wants to go but nothing happens."

What You Can Do to Help

There are some things you can do to manage a constipation problem:

- help relieve constipation
- help prevent constipation in the future

Relieve constipation

Give oral laxatives that have stool softeners in them and use them every day. Start with two at night. Add two after breakfast if there is no relief. Continue taking two to four laxative tablets every day.

Laxatives relieve constipation by stimulating the bowels to move waste products out of the body. Stool softeners draw water into the bowel and decrease the dryness of stools so stool moves down the long intestinal tract more easily. The combination of both laxatives and stool softeners gives the best results. Tablets can be bought at any pharmacy. There are many brands to choose from, but Senokot-S tablets are frequently used when constipation is caused by pain medicines. If finances are a concern, ask the pharmacist about less expensive medicines, or ask the doctor or nurse if they have office samples.

Increase the number of laxative tablets. Take three laxative tablets with stool softeners at night if the previous laxative schedule fails. Different people require different amounts of these medicines. You can increase the number of tablets to up to eight a day. People taking pain medicine may need as many as six to eight a day to prevent constipation from the pain medicine. Report side effects that are warned about on the label to a doctor or nurse immediately (for example, severe stomach cramping, nausea, or vomiting).

Give a rectal suppository after checking with the doctor or nurse. Suppositories can be inserted in the rectum, where they stimulate the lower bowel to move. Suppositories can be stored in the refrigerator since they become soft when warm. However, suppositories should not be used if the person with cancer has low platelet or white blood cell counts since there is a risk of infection or bleeding if the suppository breaks a small blood vessel in the rectal area.

Give enemas after checking with the doctor or nurse. Give a mineral oil enema, Fleets enema, or soap suds enema for immediate relief, but first check with the doctor or nurse. Enemas are the last step to try for relieving constipation. They evacuate the lower bowel, which helps the upper bowel move as well.

An oil enema softens stool. Usually, a small amount of mineral oil (four ounces) is pushed gently into the bowel through a small plastic bottle. The person then holds the oil in until feeling the urge to have a bowel movement.

A Fleets enema puts about four ounces of chemically treated (sodium phosphate or sodium biphosphate) water into the bowel along with medicines such as castor oil or laxatives.

A soap suds enema is made at home. Mix four to eight ounces of warm water with a small amount of dish soap, and then place this in a plastic enema bag. The end of the bag is lubricated with oil or Vaseline and inserted into the rectum. Then, the suds mixture is dripped slowly into the lower bowel. The bowels move because the volume of the liquid stimulates movement and because the soap suds mildly irritate the bowel.

All of these enemas and equipment can be bought at a pharmacy. There is also a small (two inches long) enema that is easy to insert and works well.

Only one or two enemas are usually needed to relieve constipation. It is best to give an enema with the person lying on his or her left side near a bathroom or with a commode next to the bed or couch.

Prevent constipation

There are many things you can do to prevent constipation. If the person with cancer has been constipated recently, then use these strategies to help prevent it in the future.

Gradually add foods high in fiber to the diet, such as:

- whole grain cereals and breads
- dried fruits such as prunes and raisins
- popcorn, nuts, and seeds
- beans and legumes
- raw fruits and vegetables

High-fiber foods draw water into the stools. They also provide bulk—that is, they are made of materials that do not break down as the food passes through the intestines, where it is normally dissolved by acids and enzymes. For example, skins and coverings on nuts, beans, grains, fruits, and vegetables are not easily broken down, and these help form stools that are easily passed out of the body. If raw fruits and vegetables are hard to chew, try grating or cooking them.

Add unprocessed bran to the diet. Bran stimulates bowel activity. Sprinkle it on cereal or mix it with yogurt, applesauce, or pudding. Start with two teaspoons per day and gradually increase this amount up to two tablespoons per day. Be careful. Adding large amounts of bran too quickly to the diet might cause gas, diarrhea, and discomfort.

Encourage the drinking of plenty of fluids, up to six to eight glasses of liquid every day. Fluids add water to the stools and prevent constipation caused by dry, hard stools.

Offer hot or warm liquids. They stimulate the bowels. People often say that coffee makes them go to the bathroom. The combination of caffeine and hot liquid causes this.

Serve prune juice, hot lemon water, or tea. Prune juice, whether warm or cold, and hot lemon water or tea all stimulate the bowels.

Encourage exercise, such as walking every day. Even a small amount of movement, such as walking in the house, helps stimulate muscles that make the bowel work. Talk to the doctor about the amount and type of exercise that is best for the person with cancer.

Avoid regular use of enemas, if possible. Enemas may prevent the intestines from finding a regular pattern.

Give one or two stool softeners every day, and use a laxative if taking opioids. One or two stool softeners every day can help prevent constipation. If the person is eating or drinking less and not feeling well enough to exercise, then try stool softeners. If opioids are taken, give a daily laxative and read the chapter *Cancer Pain* (pages 135–157) for a more complete explanation of using laxatives with opioids.

Maintain a daily schedule of prevention. First, try diet and exercise, then medicines, and follow a daily schedule just the way you do with other medicines. Following a schedule of diet, drinking liquids, exercise, and preventive medicines will add up to successful prevention.

Possible Obstacles

Here are some obstacles that others have faced in managing this problem:

"She hasn't eaten much all month. How could anything be in there to plug her up or make her constipated?"

The body makes waste products and stool even when people eat very little. Taking narcotics (opioids), not walking much, or not drinking enough fluids also makes constipation more likely to happen. Laxatives and sometimes enemas are needed to get the bowels moving.

"He's too embarrassed about his constipation to tell me about it—so how can I help him?"

Put him in charge of his own care. Have him read this chapter. If possible, help him to understand what causes constipation and what to do about it. Then he can be responsible for managing it. Another strategy is to have him talk directly to a nurse. Most people are willing to talk about "embarrassing" things to health professionals. Also, health professionals are experienced in discussing these subjects without embarrassment.

Think of other obstacles that could interfere with carrying out your plan

What additional roadblocks could get in the way of doing the things recommended in this chapter? For example, will the person with cancer cooperate? Will other people help? How will you explain your needs to other people? Do you have the time and energy to carry out the plan?

Develop plans for getting around these roadblocks using the six problem-solving steps discussed in the first section of this book (see pages xi–xvi).

Carrying Out and Adjusting Your Plan

Carrying out your plan

Prepare in advance for constipation, especially if narcotics (opioids) are prescribed or if the person is less active. Use this chapter as a reference and begin to change diet and food habits to prevent constipation.

Checking on results

After new medicines are started, ask the person with cancer if bowel habits are changing. Ask if the constipation is happening less frequently. When does it happen? Do you both know what to do to relieve it? Are actions to prevent constipation taking effect?

If your plan doesn't work...

If your plan does not seem to be working or constipation is getting worse, consider the following:

- Check the *When to Get Professional Help* section (pages 166–168). If you observe any of the listed conditions, call the doctor or nurse.
- Review the strategies in the section *What You Can Do to Help* (pages 168–171) to be sure you are doing everything you can to deal with this problem.
- If constipation continues, ask the doctor or nurse for help. Tell them what you have done and what the results have been.

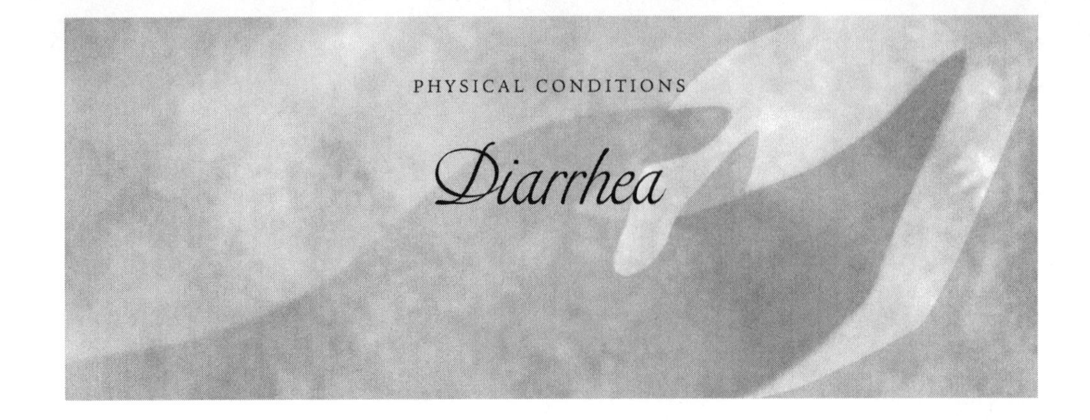

Understanding the Condition

Diarrhea is defined as liquid stools. With diarrhea, bowel movements can happen more frequently and feel more urgent. Having diarrhea can also be very upsetting. It can be caused by cancer treatments, cancer medicines, other medicines, and sometimes emotional distress. Losing fluids through diarrhea adds to fatigue and feeling "washed out." Diarrhea can also cause dehydration, which can be a serious health problem. Therefore, stopping diarrhea is important for both comfort and health. Another possible side effect of diarrhea is a rectal infection. Rectal infections can be caused by bacteria that invade the body when the skin is broken from the acids and irritants in the diarrhea stool. This is uncomfortable and painful.

Diarrhea can have serious health effects, so correct management is important. Be especially alert for dehydration. Get professional help early for severe diarrhea and encourage drinking fluids. If the person is unable to take care of him or herself, you will have to deal with the diarrhea directly, which can be very stressful—especially if it continues for a long time. This is when you will need help from others.

Your goals are to:

- call for professional help when it is needed
- insure that medicines to prevent diarrhea are taken correctly
- replace lost fluids and nutrients after diarrhea
- discourage eating foods that make diarrhea worse
- do what you can to increase comfort

When to Get Professional Help

All of these "call now" problems demand quick attention because there is a danger that too much fluid is being lost. Serious health problems can result if a person is dehydrated for a long time.

Call the doctor or nurse if any of the following conditions exist:

- **Severe diarrhea.** Severe diarrhea means a lot of fluid is being lost. With severe diarrhea, stools are very runny, and the person often complains of stomach cramps as well. The severity of the problem depends on many factors, such as the person's weight or previous state of fluid balance.

  Losing small amounts of fluid and stool in diarrhea can be dangerous for a small, thin person or for anyone who has recently been struggling with diarrhea or vomiting. In this situation, dehydration happens quickly. Reporting severe diarrhea early is important so medicines and fluids can be given to stop the diarrhea and to reverse or correct the dehydration.

- **Diarrhea for more than one day.**
- **Blood in the diarrhea stool.**
- **Fever 100.5°F or above with diarrhea.**

Know the following facts before you call the doctor or nurse:

- How many bowel movements are usual each day?____________
- How many bowel movements have there been in the last 24 hours?

  ____
- How runny were they? ______________________________
- Are there any other symptoms with the diarrhea?____________

  ____stomach pain

  ____stomach cramps

  ____bloating (feeling very full in the stomach or abdomen)

  ____nausea (sick to the stomach)

____vomiting

____fever

____bloody diarrhea

- How much liquid was taken and how much was eaten in the last two days? ______________________

  Knowing the approximate amounts of liquids and foods taken helps the doctor and nurse know if the body is receiving enough to replace what is being lost. Dehydration is important to treat because it could lead to dangerously low blood pressure and chemical imbalance in the body. Sometimes IV fluids are ordered to balance the fluid loss and put important fluids, water, vitamins, and minerals back into the body.

- What medicines were taken in the last two to three days? At what dosage?

  ____chemotherapy (when?) ______________________

  ____laxatives ______________________

  ____antidiarrhea tablets or liquids ______________________

  ____other medicines including nonprescription and herbal medicines ______________________

- Has weight been lost? How much? ______________________
- Is there any history of other bowel problems, such as diverticulitis, colitis, or irritable bowel syndrome? ______________________

What You Can Do to Help

There are several things you can do to manage this problem:

- give medicines for diarrhea
- replace lost fluids and nutrients
- avoid certain foods
- increase comfort

Give medicines for diarrhea

Antidiarrhea medicine is a fast way to stop this problem. These medicines slow down the bowel.

Check with the doctor or nurse before you give antidiarrhea medicines that can be bought without a prescription. The doctor might prefer that you use a prescription medicine or certain over-the-counter (non-prescription) drugs to stop diarrhea.

Follow the instructions on the bottle or on the prescription. Sometimes antidiarrhea medicines do the job too well. If too much is given, they can cause cramping and constipation. The person may get very sleepy if given too much antidiarrhea medicine.

Replace lost fluids and nutrients

Important fluids are lost with diarrheal stool. Replacing them is crucial. Try to increase fluid intake to three quarts a day—unless the doctor or nurse says otherwise. Here are several ways to do this:

Offer clear liquids, for example, chicken broth; weak, tepid tea; apple, cranberry, or grape juice; ginger ale; Jell-O; Popsicles; and Gatorade. They provide important nutrients but also let the bowel rest. Clear liquids are easier for the intestines to absorb into the bloodstream, and they help replace the fluids being lost with diarrhea.

Serve fluids between meals. Drinking fluids between meals keeps a steady amount of water and other nutrients entering the body. Drinking between meals is less likely to cramp a sore stomach or intestines.

Serve low-fiber foods, for example, bananas, rice, applesauce, mashed potatoes, dry toast, crackers, eggs, fish, poultry, cottage cheese, and yogurt. Low-fiber foods do not attract or pull water out of the body into the bowel. They are easier to digest than high-fiber vegetables.

Serve small meals throughout the day instead of three larger meals. Try six small meals in a day. Smaller meals are easier to digest and the total amount of food or liquid taken in is often larger with frequent small meals than with three large meals.

Increase high-potassium foods in the diet, such as apricot or peach nectar, bananas, and mashed or baked potatoes. People tend to lose potassium when they have diarrhea. This chemical is vital to the body and needs to be replaced.

Avoid certain foods

Some foods increase the action of the bowel and how quickly it pulls fluid out of body tissues into stool. Avoiding these foods helps to reduce problems with diarrhea.

Avoid serving foods that produce gas, such as beans, raw vegetables, raw fruits, broccoli, corn, cabbage, cauliflower, carbonated drinks, and chewing gum. These foods cause a feeling of fullness and makes a person stop eating or drinking earlier. Gas also adds to discomfort. Avoid chewing gum because it makes some people swallow air, which also adds to abdominal discomfort.

Avoid serving foods that contain acids, such as citrus juices like orange or grapefruit. These make the stomach and intestines churn and can create more discomfort as well as more diarrhea.

Avoid serving fat, such as fatty meats and greasy fried foods. Fats are difficult to digest. If the person has diarrhea, fats are pushed through the intestines without being digested. Undigested fat increases the amount and frequency of diarrhea.

Cool down hot food or hot drinks. Hot foods and liquids make the bowels move. Avoid these until the diarrhea has ended.

Limit caffeine intake, for example, coffee, strong teas, sodas with caffeine, and chocolate. Caffeine makes the bowel work faster. If a person has diarrhea, you want to slow down his or her bowels, which are already overactive.

Avoid giving milk and milk products if they seem to make diarrhea worse. Milk can make diarrhea worse. It can also cause stomach cramps in some adults.

Increase comfort

The lower abdomen can become quite sore from intestinal cramps that may accompany diarrhea. The person with cancer can also feel worn out from bouts with diarrhea. Rectal skin or skin around a stoma (an opening in the skin on the abdomen for stool to come out into a bag) can become very sore. There are several ways to ease abdominal or skin soreness. Encourage the person with diarrhea to do the following:

Put a warm water bottle wrapped in a towel on the abdomen. Warmth on the stomach can relieve pain and discomfort caused by stomach tightness or cramps. However, do not use a heating pad or very hot water in the water bottle. The skin may be sensitive to heat, especially if the person is receiving chemotherapy or radiation therapy, and a heating pad or very hot water bottle could cause skin problems.

Cleanse the rectal area. After diarrhea, cleanse the outside of the rectum gently with warm water and then dry the skin to reduce redness and prevent infection. Always clean the rectal area from the front to the back so stool will not be spread towards the opening to the bladder or vagina.

Soak in warm water. Use a tub or Sitz bath. Sitz baths can be bought at most pharmacies or medical equipment stores. Sitz baths are plastic bowls that are placed over the toilet; the person can sit in the bowl of warm water while it spills into the toilet below. Sitting in a tub of warm water can also be helpful.

Apply soothing creams, ointments, or astringent pads such as Tucks to the rectal area. Creams prevent rectal skin from chapping in the same way they prevent diaper rash or chapping on infants' skin. Try brands such as Nupercainal, A&D, or Vaseline. Astringent pads also help dry the area and soothe irritated skin.

If diarrhea continues and the rectal area becomes very sore and red, apply an ointment such as Desitin to protect the skin. Fluids will be less likely to burn the skin since this type of ointment covers the skin with a protective layer.

Protect the bed and chairs from being soiled by putting two overlapping waterproof pads or Chux (also called blue pads) under the buttocks where the person will lie or sit. For the bed, a plastic trash bag under the Chux will give extra protection as will a plastic mattress pad.

Talk to an enterostomal therapy nurse for recommendations if the person with cancer has a stoma and the skin around the opening becomes irritated.

Possible Obstacles

Think about what might prevent you from controlling or preventing diarrhea.

Here is one obstacle that other people have faced:

"He's had nothing to eat or drink for days, so this diarrhea can't last much longer."

The body can keep removing fluid for much longer than you think. The fluid is drawn from body tissues, and diarrhea can continue even if the person stops eating or drinking for days. It's important to replace the fluids that are lost even if the person thinks these will be washed out instantly.

Think of other obstacles that could interfere with carrying out your plan

What additional roadblocks could get in the way of doing the things recommended in this chapter? For example, will the person with cancer cooperate? Will other people help? How will you explain your needs to other people? Do you have the time and energy to carry out the plan?

Develop plans for getting around these roadblocks using the six problem-solving steps discussed in the first section of this book (see pages xi–xvi).

Carrying Out and Adjusting Your Plan

Checking on results

Keep track of the frequency and severity of diarrhea. Are you able to stop the diarrhea when it starts? Is the rectal skin or skin around a stoma well cared for and protected? Are other precautions with fluids and diet being followed to prevent diarrhea?

If your plan doesn't work...

If problems with diarrhea are getting worse or the person with cancer is becoming worn out, review the section *When to Get Professional Help* (pages 175–176). When calling, tell the doctor or nurse what was done to deal with diarrhea and discuss what else can be done.

If diarrhea isn't severe but continues for several days, ask the doctor or nurse for help. Tell them what you have done and what the results have been.

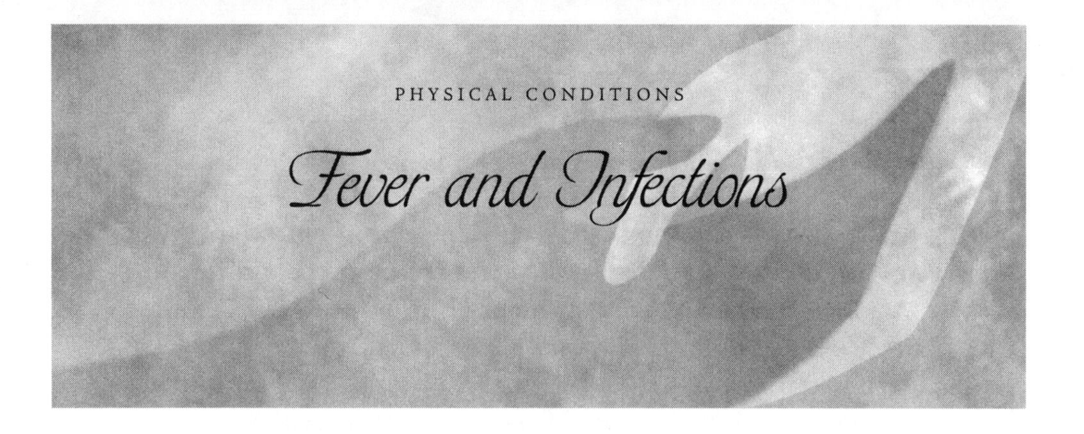

Understanding the Condition

There are a few special things to keep in mind about fevers during cancer treatments. First, they can happen very easily and they can get out of hand easily too. So it's important to be on the lookout for fevers and act quickly to keep them under control. Dehydration is something to be especially alert for since it can result in a visit to the emergency room. Second, there is a lot you can do to prevent fevers in someone receiving chemotherapy or radiation therapy. This chapter has many lists of things to do. Managing fevers takes organization—and the lists will help you stay organized.

Some chemotherapies or radiation therapies increase the chances of getting infections—usually for a short time following treatments. This happens when the treatments reduce the white blood cell count, which leaves the person at a higher risk of infection. This condition is called neutropenia.

If signs of infection such as swelling, pain, or redness occur when the white blood cell count is low, it is important to treat the cause of these problems immediately. Take action before a high temperature develops. The body cannot fight infection well when the number of white blood cells is low—early action is the key. If the problem is severe, the doctor may order a medicine to increase the number of white blood cells.

Fever is another sign of a possible infection. Fevers can be tiring, and the chills that may come with fevers can be frightening and exhausting. A very high fever can also be dangerous. Antibiotic medicines are often needed, at least until the number of white blood cells is back to normal.

Your goals are to:

- call for professional help if it is needed
- lower fevers after reporting them
- reduce the chance of future fevers and infections

When to Get Professional Help

Call the doctor, nurse, or the after-hours telephone number right away (no matter what time it is) for any of the following conditions:

- **A temperature of 100.5°F or higher by mouth.** A temperature of 98.6°F is normal for most people. Any higher temperature is a fever. Temperatures of 100.5°F and higher usually indicate a problem requiring medical help. (If the person with cancer's normal temperature is different from 98.6°F, ask the doctor or nurse what temperature indicates a fever. This is usually two degrees above the person's normal temperature.)

  Buy a new thermometer if you have one you don't trust or can't read. A digital thermometer is the easiest to use. It lights up and shows you the exact temperature when it is finished recording. Digital thermometers take the guess work out of deciding if a person has a fever. Ask your pharmacist or a store clerk to help you select one. Don't use a rectal thermometer unless your doctor or nurse approves its use. If the platelet count is low, the delicate tissue in the rectum may bleed when a thermometer is inserted.

- **Severe shaking chills that last 20 minutes or more.** Chills happen before a temperature rises. Take the temperature when the chills are over and the shaking has stopped.

- **Frequent, painful urination.** Pain with urination usually indicates a urinary infection. People with this type of infection urinate in very small amounts. They also feel the urge to urinate even though little urine is in the bladder. When they do urinate, a sharp pain shoots through the lower abdomen and they may have a burning sensation.

- **No urine output for six to eight hours.** It's important to report if the person has not urinated in the past day. This condition has many different possible causes, including infections, and needs to be investigated.

- **New cough, shortness of breath, or rapid breathing.** Report any problems with breathing or coughing, especially a feeling that it is hard to draw air into the lungs or to release air. Labored or difficult breathing could be caused by an infection, and should be reported even if the person doesn't have a fever.

- ▲ **Changes in mental status.** Cloudy thinking or mild confusion may be a sign of infection and should be reported.

When symptoms are not an emergency, but should be reported

Some symptoms are not an emergency but should be reported during regular office or clinic hours. Call if any of the following conditions exist.

Too weak to drink fluids. Drinking fluids is important for a person with fever. When the person's temperature rises, the body loses water that needs to be replaced. If it is not replaced, the person may become dehydrated. Fevers may cause severe fatigue, which makes it hard to drink. Therefore, when you report a fever, tell how much liquid the person has been drinking.

Any new redness or swelling on the skin or at an IV or injection site. Skin redness or swelling may also indicate an infection. When the white blood cell counts are low, small cuts or scrapes can easily become infected.

Cold symptoms (runny nose, stuffy nose, watery eyes) or sore throat. Infections develop quickly in the mouth or throat. Report cold symptoms, even when there is no fever.

New sinus, abdominal, or back pain. New pains in these areas may be the result of a new infection or the spread of an old infection.

Toothache. Infections in the mouth or gums can cause toothaches. Antibiotics are often prescribed to prevent infection around the tooth. Dental work should be postponed until enough antibiotics are in the bloodstream to fight infection. Check with the doctor treating the infection before any invasive dental work is scheduled.

Aching and lack of energy that doesn't go away. These symptoms may be the result of a low-grade infection.

Know the following facts before calling the doctor or nurse:

- How many hours has the fever been higher than 100.5°F (by mouth)? ______________________________

  You may not know exactly how long the temperature has been high. Report the time that you took the temperature and the time you first noticed any other changes, such as redder skin, more sweating, or complaints about feeling hot or feverish.

- How much liquid did the person with fever drink in the last eight hours or since the fever began, and how much urine was passed?

  ____

  This tells the doctor or nurse if dehydration (not having enough water in the body) from fever is becoming serious.

- Has the person with cancer had other fevers since cancer treatments began? ______________________________
  - How many fevers? ______________________________
  - When have they occurred? ______________________________
  - After how many chemotherapy, radiation, or other cancer treatments did they begin? ______________________________

  If there has been a pattern of fevers after chemotherapy in the past, give this information when you call.

- What medicines has the person taken to lower fever or fight infections (for example, acetaminophen [Tylenol] or antibiotics)? When were they last taken? ______________________________

  ____

- When was the last cancer treatment, what was it, and what were the names of any drugs given? ______________________________

  ____

  Some drugs create mild reactions for a short time. The doctor or nurse can judge what is normal for the drugs that were given.

- What were the most recent blood counts, and what date were the blood samples drawn? ______________________________

Here is an example of what you might say when calling about a fever or infection:

"My mother is Dr. Harvey's patient. She's had shaking chills for more than 20 minutes. Then I took her temperature and it was 101.6°F. She had chemotherapy last week. What should I do?"

What You Can Do to Help

There are some things you can do at home to deal with a fever:

- reduce the fever after reporting it
- prevent fever and infection

Reduce the fever after reporting it

Certain medicines lower fevers. These drugs do not remove what caused the fever, but they do help lower the temperature and make the person feel better.

Give acetaminophen (adult dose) unless you have been told not to give it. Acetaminophen (Tylenol and other brands) lowers body temperature. It also fights swelling and soreness and makes the person with cancer feel more comfortable. Acetaminophen does not make fever disappear, but it lowers the temperature and reduces the side effects of fever such as fatigue or aching.

Give any medicines for fever or infection prescribed by your doctor.

Put cold washcloths on the forehead if the person with cancer is hot. Cooling the forehead lowers the discomfort of feeling very hot. In addition, the cool cloths cool the blood that flows through the head close to the surface of the skin.

Encourage drinking two to three quarts of cool liquid over a 12-hour period, unless large amounts of fluid are not allowed. The body needs more fluid when feverish because more fluids than usual are being lost through the skin and lungs. The person with fever runs the risk of dehydration when the fever is high. Drinking fluids replaces lost water.

Serve high-calorie, high-carbohydrate foods such as pasta, bread, fruit, potatoes, and energy bars. The body's metabolism increases with fever. This means that the person with fever is burning calories at a faster rate than normal. High-calorie, high-carbohydrate foods replace the nutrients that are being burned up and help restore some of the lost energy.

Change damp clothing and bed linens. When the person with fever sweats, moisture dries on the skin. This is uncomfortable and can also make the body cool down rapidly, causing shaking and chills.

Do not overdress the person with a fever. Do not pile on blankets or turn up the heat since this can increase the fever, which could cause more health problems.

Prevent fever and infection

Here are some ways to prevent infections:

Encourage the person with cancer to wash their hands frequently, especially before preparing food, before eating, after using the bathroom, and when tending another sick person, a baby, or a pet. Hand washing is the best way to limit the spread of germs. People with cancer can get infections from their own skin, mouth, and tissues. They can also get infections from others. Wash the skin and hands frequently and brush the teeth at least three times a day to wash away potentially dangerous germs.

Encourage using lotions and moisturizers on the skin to keep the skin moist and to prevent drying, chapping, and cracking. Bacteria can enter dry skin cracks and start an infection.

Avoid sharing unwashed thermometers, toothbrushes, or drinking glasses. Anything that goes in the mouth, including forks, spoons, or dinner knives, can pass germs from one person to another if not washed.

Avoid taking rectal temperatures. These cannot be compared to oral temperatures, which are the ones usually recorded on the medical chart. Also, taking a rectal temperature adds to the risk of infection because the thermometer may cut or injure membranes inside the rectum. If it is not possible to obtain an oral temperature, place the thermometer under the person's armpit. This is known as taking the axillary temperature.

Ask people with colds or who are ill to wait to visit until they are better.

Avoid raw fruit and vegetables that are not washed, raw or undercooked eggs, and food handled by others, when the white blood cell count is low. People with low white blood cell counts have difficulty warding off infections caught from others, and food is a common carrier of germs from other people. Washing (or cooking) fruits and vegetables before eating them removes many germs. Deli items, which are already sliced, cannot usually be washed, so it's wise to buy and slice meats and cheeses yourself until white blood cell counts are higher, and the risk of infection is lower.

Offer liquids to prevent urinary infections. Urinary infections are less likely to happen when the kidneys, bladder, and urinary system are flushed with water. Avoid caffeine and alcohol because these irritate the opening where the urine comes out and can break open the skin in that area. Encourage drinking about three quarts of liquid each day.

Encourage good dental hygiene, including tooth brushing after eating and soaking dentures daily.

Replace toothbrushes every three months. Toothbrushes harbor bacteria and other organisms because they are wet most of the time. Replace them at least every three months to reduce the chance of infection in the mouth.

Get a new toothbrush after treating a mouth infection (usually a thrush infection).

Recommend thoroughly cleaning the rectal area after bowel movements. Women should cleanse the rectal area from front to back. This motion is less likely to cause a urinary infection because you are wiping away from the opening where urine comes out.

For women, recommend using sanitary pads and not tampons during menstrual periods. Tampons breed bacteria more easily and can cause tears in the vagina that lead to infection.

Thoroughly wash skin that is not open to the air, such as the skin in the groin area and underneath the breasts. Air these areas for a short time after washing to be sure they are dry.

Encourage wearing shoes to prevent cuts and bruises. Even small cuts on the feet can allow bacteria into the body. Cuts do not heal quickly when the white blood cell count is low.

Wash cuts right away with soap and water.

Encourage using a sunscreen lotion and staying out of the sun between 10:00 A.M. and 4:00 P.M. Sunburn leads to blisters and splits the skin open. Once the skin is open, it's easier for bacteria to enter the body.

Arrange for someone other than the person with cancer to groom pets, empty cat litter boxes, and clean pet cages. Pet feces contain many bacteria and fungi, which are easily transferred to a person with a low white blood cell count. It is best to have someone else clean the pets until the white blood cell count of the person with cancer returns to a normal level.

Possible Obstacles

Here are some obstacles that other people have faced:

"High fevers burn up whatever is causing the problem."

High fevers are dangerous and should be reported and taken care of. These conditions can lead to dehydration and seizures. High temperatures do not burn up the bacteria that are causing the problem.

"I've had fevers before, and they didn't last long. It will go away by itself."

When the white blood cell count is low, fevers will not disappear on their own. Fevers can be serious and should be reported and treated. If they are not, the temperature may rise too high and may lead to dehydration. Avoid high temperatures and report any possible signs of infection whether or not a fever occurs with them.

"I didn't know I had a fever."

If your body feels warm, aches, or feels like the flu, take your temperature. If it is above normal, reread this chapter for what to do.

Think of other obstacles that could interfere with carrying out your plan

What additional roadblocks could get in the way of doing the things recommended in this chapter? For example, will the person with cancer cooperate? Will other people help? How will you explain your needs to other people? Do you have the time and energy to carry out the plan?

Develop plans for getting around these roadblocks using the six problem-solving steps discussed in the first section of this book (see pages xi–xvi).

Carrying Out and Adjusting Your Plan

Checking on results

Keep records of when fevers happen so you can see if they are occurring more or less often. Check regularly that the person with cancer is avoiding situations that increase the risk of his or her getting an infection.

If your plan doesn't work...

If fever remains a problem, or if fevers are happening more often check the *When to Get Professional Help* section (pages 182–184) to see if you need to call the doctor or nurse immediately. If fever problems continue, ask the doctor or nurse for help. Tell them what you have done and what the results have been.

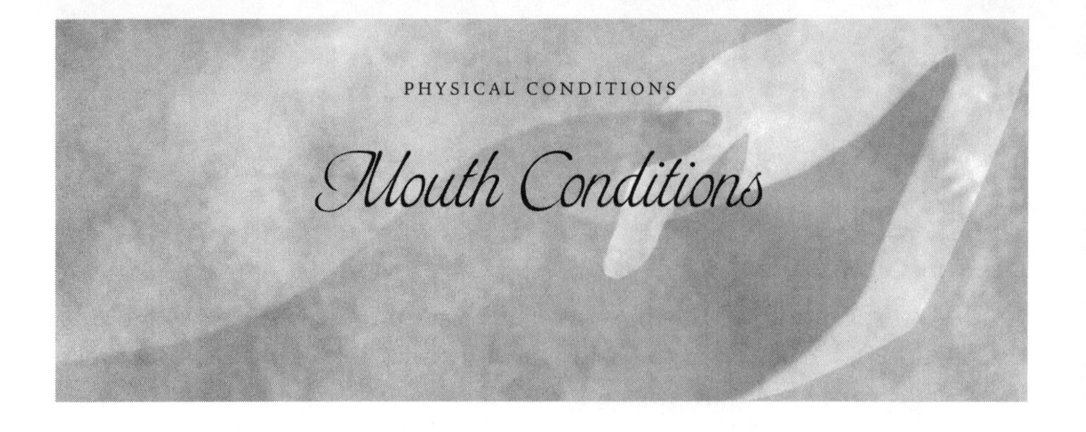

Understanding the Condition

Mouth problems associated with cancer treatments can be very painful and can interfere with eating. This chapter tells how to deal with this difficult problem and, equally important, it tells what you can do to prevent mouth problems.

Problems with the mouth are a common side effect of cancer treatments because the skin inside of the mouth contains rapidly growing cells. Chemotherapy can slow the growth of healthy cells in the mouth. As a result, the mouth tissues are weakened, mouth sores develop, and sores take longer to heal.

Cancer and cancer treatments can temporarily reduce the ability of a person's immune system to fight infection. When the immune system cannot protect the body from normal bacteria or outside germs, weakened or inflamed tissues in the mouth can become infected. A sore and tender throat and esophagus (the tube leading to the stomach) can also develop. Sometimes the doctor will prescribe a medicine to boost the person's immune system.

Your goals are to:

- call for professional help when it is needed
- treat any mouth sores, ulcers, or infections
- do what you can to prevent mouth problems

When to Get Professional Help

Report the signs and symptoms listed below to the doctor or nurse. They can then determine if an infection is beginning in the mouth, tongue, throat, or esophagus. Sometimes these problems become so severe the person must take pain medication or be hospitalized for antibiotic therapy.

Call the doctor or nurse if any of the following conditions exist:

- ▲ **Temperature more than 100.5°F.** Fever can indicate a mouth infection. If the temperature goes up suddenly, report it. However, a mouth infection can occur before the temperature goes up, so fever is not the only thing to watch for.

- ▲ **A light redness on the tongue gets much redder.** Redness comes before a mouth sore. You will need a light to tell if the mouth, gums, or tongue are redder than usual. Use a small flashlight to look into the mouth and find sores. Check the mouth twice a day, morning and night. Look at the roof of the mouth and all of the lining. Look under the tongue and gums. If the person wears dentures, remove them before checking the mouth.

- ▲ **Redness on tongue turns to white patches or white patches appear on gums or in mouth.** White patches indicate an infection. Usually it's a thrush infection (called *Candida albicans*). This infection occurs when the lining in the mouth is unable to fight off normal bacteria, and, as a result, bacteria increase in number and become a problem.

- ▲ **Complaint of "cotton" mouth or a very thick feeling on the tongue when rubbed against upper teeth.** A cottony feeling in the mouth or on the tongue also means an infection may be starting. Call and report this right away.

- ▲ **A sore or an ulcer on the lips or in the mouth.** If the normal skin covering the mouth is changed by chemotherapy, mouth soreness and sometimes mouth sores or ulcers follow.

- ▲ **Sore throat or painful throat.** The lining of the throat is the same as the lining of the mouth. The throat is just as likely to get red and sore as the mouth is.

- ▲ **So much difficulty swallowing that medicine is not being taken as often as prescribed.** Trouble with swallowing may prevent taking medicine. When the throat is sore or swollen, swallowing becomes more difficult. Call if medicines are skipped because swallowing is too painful.
- ▲ **So much difficulty swallowing or drinking and eating that little food or fluid is taken for two days.** The person with cancer may be eating or drinking less because of a sore or painful throat. This can cause weakness and possibly dehydration. Treatment for mouth soreness will help with eating and drinking.

Know the following facts before you call the doctor or nurse:

- When did the mouth problems start?__________
- Is the mouth, tongue, or throat redder than usual? __________
- Are there white patches in the mouth?__________
- What was eaten and how many liquids were taken in the past 48 hours?__________
- How are the mouth and teeth cleaned? Are any special rinses used to prevent mouth sores? __________
- Is the person with cancer smoking or using an oral tobacco product? If yes, how much?__________
- Was any alcohol taken? If yes, how much?__________
- Is there a change in chewing or swallowing? __________
- Has any medicine been ordered for the mouth or throat? If so, how often is it taken?__________
- Do any medicines for the mouth cause problems such as gagging or nausea so they are taken less often than prescribed?__________
- When was the last radiation or chemotherapy treatment, and what chemotherapy drugs were given? Have there been any recent changes in treatments?__________
- Is the person taking any treatments not prescribed by a doctor such as herbs or vitamins?__________

Here is an example of what you might say when calling:

"My sister is Dr. Smith's patient. She has a cottony feeling in her mouth. Also, her throat hurts so badly that she is only taking the medicine once a day that was prescribed for four times a day."

What You Can Do to Help

Here are some things you can do to help deal with mouth sores or a sore mouth:

- moisten a dry mouth
- soothe a sore mouth and ease swallowing
- treat mouth sores, ulcers, or infections
- prevent mouth problems

Moisten a dry mouth

Dry mouth is a frequent side effect of medicines taken for cancer. A dry mouth makes it harder to chew and swallow. There are several ways to help a dry mouth. Encourage the person with a dry mouth to do the following:

Rinse the mouth before meals and throughout the day. Rinsing the mouth helps to moisten it and remove the feeling of being parched or dry. Don't use rinses that have alcohol in them because they dry the mouth.

Use a lip moisturizer before eating. If the lips are moist, food is easier to chew and enjoy. Put a thin coat of petroleum jelly, lip salve, or cocoa butter on the lips.

Drink small sips of liquids with meals.

Sip two to three quarts of liquid a day, unless large amounts of fluid are not allowed.

Eat ice chips, Popsicles, frozen juices, or frozen drinks. They provide liquids and can be quite refreshing. The sugar content in Popsicles also makes the mouth water, which decreases dryness.

Dunk bread, crackers, and baked foods in coffee, tea, milk, or soup to make them moist. Moistening food makes it easier to chew and swallow. Dip bread in soup, shredded meat in marinade, or toast in coffee.

Mix gravies, sauces, salad dressings, melted butter or margarine, mayonnaise, or yogurt into food. Sauces and gravies are good ways to moisten food. They can be added toward the end of cooking or when food is reheated.

Eat soft, liquid foods. These include applesauce, canned fruits, casseroles, cooked cereal, baby foods, Popsicles, custard, cottage cheese, bananas, puddings, ice cream, gelatin, sherbet, yogurt, milk shakes, soups, stews, watermelon, and seedless grapes. If the food is not liquid to begin with, grind it or put it in a blender. Many people with cancer use blenders to enjoy foods they cannot chew easily. Even a steak can be tenderized and pureed and all of the good flavor remains.

Ask about artificial saliva. Bottles of artificial saliva can be ordered through most pharmacies. It comes in a bottle and is made of glycerin, purified water, and a few other ingredients. Xerolube, Mouthkote, or Salivert are examples of commercial products that are available in a mint flavor. There are also gum products available, such as Biotene gum, that stimulate saliva.

Soothe a sore mouth and ease swallowing

Some chemotherapy causes mouth sores, which make eating and swallowing difficult. Here are things you can encourage the person with cancer to do for this problem:

Rinse the mouth with baking soda after eating, using a solution of ½ teaspoon of baking soda in 1 cup of tap water. Salt or baking soda, or both, soothes the mouth and helps it heal. Rinsing after eating removes food particles that could irritate the gums, but it does so more gently than commercial mouthwashes, many of which contain alcohol that dries out the mouth.

Drink plenty of liquids and suck on ice chips.

Use a blender or hand masher to soften foods. Softer foods are easier to chew and swallow. They are less likely to tear any sores or scrape raw tissues.

Moisten food with cream, cottage cheese, ricotta cheese, milk, gravy, and sauces. Moist food is easier to swallow, especially when the mouth and throat are tender.

Drink pureed food from a cup or through a straw. Soft food can be liquefied in a blender and poured into a cup for drinking. Using a straw helps the liquid bypass some of the sore mouth tissue when eating. Many proteins and calories can be taken in this way. If the person is too weak to use a straw, then fill the straw with an inch or two of liquid and drop the liquid in the mouth slowly.

Eat soft, moist, bland foods. These include soups, eggs, pastas, quiches, cottage cheese, ricotta cheese, tofu, tempeh, baby foods, cheese dishes, tuna fish, applesauce, custards, pudding, canned fruit, cooked cereals, bananas, gelatin, yogurt, ice cream, sherbet, frozen fruit bars, Popsicles, or shakes.

Treat mouth sores, ulcers, or infections

Encourage the person with cancer to use the following list at the first hint of a mouth sore or infection to reduce the seriousness of mouth and throat infections.

Rinse the mouth with warm tap water after eating or drinking, or use any of these:

- ½ teaspoon of salt in 2 cups of water
- ½ teaspoon of baking soda in 1 cup of water
- ½ teaspoon of salt and ½ teaspoon of baking soda in 2 cups of water

Mouth rinses remove food particles that may build up and cause bacteria to grow. Rinses also soothe sore tissues and help them heal faster. Rinse at least four times a day and as often as every two hours while awake, if possible. If the salt rinse burns, use the baking soda recipe or use less salt.

Ask about using a numbing liquid to use as a "throat coat" before eating and swallowing. Many people swallow mouth gels or "throat coats" (a thick jelly-like liquid) before meals and at bedtime when the mouth is very sore because of chemotherapy. This medicine numbs the tongue and throat enough to let liquid and soft foods pass without much trouble. The medicine also usually contains Maalox and liquid Benadryl, which heal and soothe the soreness and decrease swelling and inflammation, especially in the throat and esophagus. Ask about these mouth gels or medicines if they haven't been prescribed as part of the chemotherapy.

Another type of soothing medicine (called a "slurry") comes in tablet form and dissolves in water. It works quickly to remove any burning feeling and helps to heal the lining of the mouth and throat. Report to the doctor if the person is having trouble swallowing liquid medicines for the mouth and not using them as often as prescribed. The doctor may order another type of mouth treatment.

Use a topical ointment on mouth sores to soothe pain or soreness. Some mouth sores cause so much pain they prevent the person from eating and chewing. Coating the sores with a topical ointment, such as Ambesol, numbs them long enough to help with eating. They can also relieve pain for a while when not eating.

Use a straw to sip beverages. With a straw, the person can bypass sore spots in the mouth and drink without pain.

Ask about prescription mouth rinses to swish and swallow. During chemotherapy and a few weeks after treatment, many people use a prescription mouth rinse to swish and swallow at least four times per day. This prevents infection and eases soreness.

Finish liquid antibiotics when they are prescribed to treat an infection. The doctor may order an oral liquid antibiotic. Antibiotics are ordered to kill the mouth infection. If they are effective, the person's mouth should feel better and eating and drinking should be easier in a few days. Be sure that all of the antibiotic is taken until the bottle is empty.

Ask about using mild pain pills. Mild pain medicines can be taken an hour before eating and drinking. They help reduce the pain of biting, chewing, or swallowing when the mouth feels sore or when there are mouth ulcers.

Avoid using peroxide or peroxide rinses. Peroxide kills bacteria, but it is drying. Its use can lead to a mouth and throat infection known as thrush. In rare cases, a peroxide rinse is ordered to cleanse a deep sore that is not healing. It is then followed by a gentler rinse of warm tap water. The effect lasts about four hours, so it should not be used more frequently than instructed. Do not continue using peroxide longer than seven days. If uncertain about the use of peroxide, talk with the doctor or nurse. Recent research strongly advises against using it.

Avoid glycerin swabs. These types of swabs are drying to the mucous membranes.

Eat soft foods that are easier to swallow:

- MEATS AND PROTEINS: such as beef, pork, chicken, fish, smooth peanut butter, eggs, cottage cheese, ricotta cheese, tofu, tempeh, mild cheese, macaroni and cheese, yogurt, and bean casseroles should be well cooked, tender, and easy to chew. Avoid sharp cheese, crunchy peanut butter, and spicy foods.
- VEGETABLES: include well-cooked vegetables that are easy to chew and baked or mashed potatoes. Avoid vegetables with a lot of acid such as tomatoes, potato skins, crunchy or raw vegetables, fried potatoes or vegetables, and tomato soups and sauces.
- FRUITS: include applesauce, apple juice, grape juice, nectars, prune juice, soft-cooked or fresh noncitrus fruits, and bananas. Avoid citrus fruits (such as oranges, lemons, and grapefruits) and juices and fruit peels. These contain acid that will make mouth sores hurt more.
- MILK: include milk, milk shakes, cream soups, eggnog, buttermilk, custards, and puddings.
- BREADS: include all cooked or dry soft cereals, soft bread and rolls, and pasta with mild sauce. Avoid seeded breads, crusty breads, or granola bars.

Soften breads and cereals with milk.

Mash or puree foods. Use a blender or food processor.

Use gravy, butter, or cream sauces, which add liquid to food and make it easier to swallow.

Eat foods at room temperature. Avoid extremely hot or cold foods.

Let carbonation or fizz escape from sodas.

Serve gelatin, pudding, sherbets, and softened ice cream. These foods count as liquids. They are important to offer because the person with mouth sores needs many fluids to combat a dry, sore mouth and throat to prevent dehydration and imbalances of important body chemistry.

Ask about high-calorie liquids, such as Ensure, Isocal, or milk shake recipes. You may also wish to offer these high-calorie drinks in between meals or after meals.

Avoid cigarettes, pipes, chewing tobacco, and alcoholic beverages. They will make mouth sores worse.

Prevent mouth sores

Encourage the person with cancer to:

Brush their teeth at least every four hours. Rinse their mouth every two hours with a salt water or baking soda rinse. See page 195 for mixtures. Swish with warm water for at least one minute and then spit out the rinse. Rinsing, even with warm water, removes bacteria and food buildup that can lead to mouth infections and sores. To be effective, the whole mouth care routine should take at least five minutes.

Use any of these to clean the teeth: soft toothbrush, soft sponge applicator, cotton-tipped applicator, and/or a finger wrapped with gauze or soft washcloth.

The mouth can be easily irritated. Softer toothbrushes prevent cutting or scraping and reduce the likelihood of infection.

Throw away toothbrushes after a mouth infection since they could start new infections. Change toothbrushes at least every two months.

Remove dentures when cleaning the mouth. Clean dentures with a toothbrush and a cleansing agent such as Peridex. Rinse dentures with salt water or plain water after cleaning.

Remove dentures when rinsing or sleeping. Dentures irritate a dry mouth. They can cause enough scraping to break the skin and start an infection, especially if they don't fit well.

Keep lips moist with a light coating of petroleum jelly, mild lip balm, or cocoa butter. If swallowing is difficult, then the mouth and lips become dry. Lip balms prevent chapping and infection.

Drink about two to three quarts of fluid each day—unless otherwise ordered.

Chew sugarless gum or use sugarless hard candies, which moisten the mouth. They increase saliva in the mouth. Sugarless products are recommended because they limit the buildup of bacteria. Taking frequent sips of water also helps. Many people carry large plastic cups with straws and drink from these frequently to keep the mouth moist.

Set a Water-Pik on the lowest setting, if one is used. Water from a Water-Pik can cause bleeding. The gums are very sensitive as a side effect of some chemotherapies, and they bleed easily.

Use dental floss at bedtime. Flossing removes food particles but can also cause small cuts. These heal during the night because no food is eaten for at least eight or 10 hours. However, avoid flossing when platelet or white blood cell counts are low to prevent infection and bleeding. Do not floss if it causes bleeding or pain.

Avoid commercial mouthwashes. Many commercial mouthwashes have alcohol in them, which is drying. Ask the nurses what works best and what mouthwashes are recommended.

Avoid glycerin or lemon juice mouth swabs. They are also drying. Avoid using them because the skin inside the mouth can crack and get infected when it's dry.

Possible Obstacles

Here are some obstacles that have sometimes stopped others from managing mouth sore problems:

"He doesn't want to quit smoking or drinking."

Both of these habits irritate the mouth. If the person on chemotherapy doesn't quit either habit, then it's even more important to do other things to take care of the mouth, such as frequent rinsing.

"It's upsetting for him to have soft or mashed foods."

Serve soft foods attractively. Add flavorings that the person likes. Encourage everyone in the family to eat the same or similar foods.

Think of other obstacles that could interfere with carrying out your plan

What additional roadblocks could get in the way of doing the things recommended in this chapter? For example, will the person with cancer cooperate? Will other people help? How will you explain your needs to other people? Do you have the time and energy to carry out the plan?

Develop plans for getting around these roadblocks using the six problem-solving steps discussed in the first section of this book (see pages xi–xvi).

Carrying Out and Adjusting Your Plan

Carrying out your plan

The most important thing you can do is to set up and follow a regular, daily schedule for treating and preventing mouth sores.

Checking on results

Check regularly with the person with cancer on how troublesome and uncomfortable the mouth sores are. Pay special attention to whether they interfere with eating.

If your plan doesn't work...

If problems with mouth soreness or swallowing are getting worse, review this chapter and ask yourself if you are doing everything you can to encourage good oral hygiene and protect the mouth and throat against soreness and infection. Tell the doctor or nurse what was done to deal with the mouth problems and discuss what else they recommend doing.

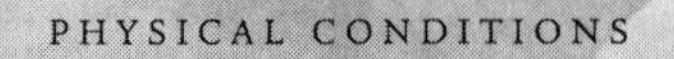

Nausea and Vomiting

Understanding the Condition

It's natural to be concerned about nausea and vomiting. They are very uncomfortable symptoms many people associate with cancer treatments. However, in the last few years, a great deal has been learned about how to control both symptoms. As a result, most people receiving treatments for cancer have much less nausea and vomiting than before.

Some people never experience any nausea or vomiting from cancer, its treatments, or other medicines. Other people deal with one or both symptoms at different times in their illness, depending on which treatments they receive and how they react to them.

Sometimes, after several treatments that have made a person nauseated, he or she may feel nauseous when seeing or smelling something associated with the treatments. For example, the smell of the treatment room or the sight of the nurse or doctor who gave the treatments may cause nausea and even vomiting. This is a normal reaction and will usually go away after treatments are over. It is a "learned" association between the sights and smells and feeling nauseous.

Your goals are to:

- call for professional help when it is needed
- make the best use of antinausea medicines
- do what you can to ease the nausea and vomiting

When to Get Professional Help

Ask the doctor or nurse to fill in the blanks below, and call them if any of the following conditions exist:

- **There is blood or "coffee ground"-looking material in the vomit.** Coffee ground-looking material is really old blood and signals that some bleeding has occurred inside the body. This happens rarely, but is important to report when it happens.
- **There is vomiting more than _____ times an hour for more than _____ hours.** Ask the doctor or nurse to help you fill in these times. For most people, vomiting three times per hour for more than twelve hours is serious, but it may be different for the person you are caring for.
- **The vomit shoots out for a distance (projectile vomiting).** Projectile vomiting may mean there are problems in the stomach or intestine that should be investigated by the doctor.
- **Two doses of any prescribed medicines are not taken or kept down because of nausea or vomiting.** Medicines will have to be given other ways until pills can stay down again.
- **Less than ___ cups of liquid are taken in 24 hours and no solid food is eaten.** Ask the doctor or nurse to help you fill this in. When vomiting, people don't drink liquids, and they may become dehydrated. Food is also needed to keep up person's energy and to fight illness. Most people need to drink more than four cups of liquid in 24 hours. Also, for most people, two days without food is dangerous. However, the needs of the person you are caring for may be different, so ask the doctor or nurse when to call about not eating or drinking.
- **Weakness or dizziness occurs with the nausea or vomiting.** It is normal to feel a little weak or dizzy with nausea, but if a person can't get up, then you need to call a doctor or nurse.
- **Severe stomach pain happens while vomiting.** Severe pain is always a reason to call the doctor immediately.

Know the following facts when you call the doctor or nurse:

- How long has nausea been a problem? ____________________
- When did it begin and how long has it lasted? ______________
  ____
- How bad was the most recent nausea? ____________________
  ____
- How much does the nausea interfere with normal activities? __
  ____
- Was medicine prescribed for nausea or vomiting? ____________
  - Name of medicine(s) __________________________________
  - How often should it be taken? __________________________
  - How many pills at one time? ___________________________
  - How many pills were taken in the last two days? ___________
  - How much relief did it give? ___________________________
  - How long did the relief last? ___________________________
- Were any nonprescription medicines taken for the nausea? If so, what were they and what were the results? _________________
  ____
- In addition to giving medicine for nausea, what was done to help the person with nausea feel better and what were the results? __
  ____
  ____
- Was the nausea followed by vomiting? ____________________
- What did the vomit look like? Was this vomit the same color as earlier vomit? If not, how was it different? _________________
  ____
- How often has vomiting happened in the last 24 hours? ______
  ____

- What other symptoms are new since the nausea or vomiting began? (Answer questions below for each new symptom.)
  - Symptom: ______________________________
  - Where in the body is it? ______________________
  - How bad is it? ___________________________
  - When did it start? _________________________
  - When does it happen? _______________________
  - How long does it last? ______________________
  - What relieves it? __________________________
  - What doesn't help? _________________________
- What and how much was eaten in the last 24 hours? _________

  ____
- What and how much liquid was taken in the last 24 hours? ____

  ____
- How frequent were bowel movements in the last two days, and were they the same amount and color as usual? Has the person taken laxatives or stool softeners recently? _______________

  ____
- What is the temperature of the person with nausea? _________
- When was the last cancer treatment, and was there anything new or different about the last treatment? ___________________

  ____

  ____

Here is an example of what you might say when calling:

"My friend is Dr. Jones' patient. She has stomach pains when she vomits. She is complaining of severe pains, and her nausea is a lot worse now."

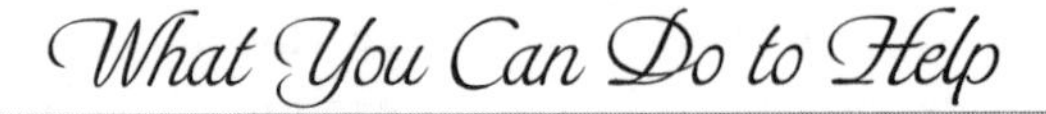

What You Can Do to Help

There are some things you can do at home to deal with a nausea or vomiting problem:

- make the best use of antinausea medicine
- learn about other ways to limit nausea and vomiting

Make the best use of antinausea medicine

Check to be sure you followed the instructions on the label (see *Appendix* on page 270) and the instructions given by the nursing staff.

Give antinausea medicine on a regular schedule. The antinausea medicine must be taken on a regular schedule to maintain enough of the medicine in the blood to be effective.

Give antinausea medicines a half hour before meals. Antinausea medicine often helps people with nausea get ready to eat and have an appetite.

Give antinausea medicine before and after receiving chemotherapy treatments. antinausea medicine should be taken before chemotherapy and then continued every four to six hours or as directed by the doctor.

A sample schedule of medicine might look like this:

- at bedtime before treatments
- in the morning before treatments
- 4 to 6 hours after treatments or as prescribed for at least 12 to 24 hours, and continue as long as nausea or vomiting persists. You can use the chart on the next page to plan when medicine should be taken (Table 5).

Other things you can do to limit nausea and vomiting

On pages 207–209 there is a list of ideas to help reduce nausea and vomiting. Start with ideas that have helped in the past, but try new ideas too. You can't be sure if something will help until you try it.

Table 5. Antinausea Medication Schedule

Mark on chart when chemotherapy treatments are scheduled and when antinausea medicine is taken.

		1:00	2:00	3:00	4:00	5:00	6:00	7:00	8:00	9:00	10:00	11:00	12:00
MONDAY	A.M.												
	P.M.												
TUESDAY	A.M.												
	P.M.												
WEDNESDAY	A.M.												
	P.M.												
THURSDAY	A.M.												
	P.M.												
FRIDAY	A.M.												
	P.M.												
SATURDAY	A.M.												
	P.M.												
SUNDAY	A.M.												
	P.M.												

Encourage eating three to four hours before treatment but not just before treatment. Eating frequent light meals during the day keeps something in the stomach and helps the body get the nutrition it needs. Try having the stomach empty just before treatments. This has helped reduce nausea for some people.

Don't serve fried foods, dairy products, and acids such as fruit juices or vinegar salad dressings. Fried and acidic foods are hard to digest and may make nausea worse.

Offer chewing gum, hard candy, or candied ginger. Try peppermint, herbal, or fruit flavors. They cover up unpleasant tastes during chemotherapy. Candied ginger can also help reduce nausea, but shouldn't be eaten in large quantities.

Let fresh air into the house or encourage the person to go outside. Taking in more oxygen helps calm the stomach and can decrease feelings of nausea. Encourage breathing through the mouth for a few minutes or open a window.

Encourage rest. Some people find it helpful to lie down when they are nauseated. Antinausea medicine often makes people sleepy, which helps them rest through their nausea. Allow short rest times between everyday activities such as dressing or walking. Taking it easy can help reduce feelings of nausea.

Offer sips of fluid two hours after vomiting. Wait a while before offering food or drink. Then offer one or two ounces of fluid at a time. Let the fizz go out of sodas before drinking them because carbonation can upset the stomach again. Stir sodas vigorously with a spoon to release carbonation, leave the can open, or leave the cap off.

Offer dry crackers. This often helps women who are pregnant and nauseated. Crackers also help many people with cancer.

Avoid unpleasant or strong odors. It may help the person with cancer to stay away from the kitchen. If odors are in the kitchen, suggest breathing through the mouth and not through the nose.

Encourage frequent mouth rinses. Frequent swishing and rinsing remove unpleasant tastes that can upset the stomach.

Suggest wearing loosely fitting clothes. Avoid tight-fitting material, especially around the waist or neck. These put pressure on the throat and stomach and add to stomach upset.

Distract attention. Watching television, listening to music, or reading may help distract the person with nausea.

Encourage relaxing. If the person with cancer is tense, physical symptoms also seem more intense. Many people find by relaxing, the symptoms are not as bothersome. (Refer to pages 98–99 for a detailed explanation of how to practice relaxation techniques.)

Encourage going with another person to treatments. A companion can show support and can help the person with cancer think and talk about other things besides the nausea and treatment. A companion can also encourage doing the relaxation exercises and even be a coach during exercises.

Possible Obstacles

Here is an obstacle that other people have faced when treating nausea:

"My husband takes medicines for other health problems that makes him sick to the stomach, and he can't stop taking those other pills. What can I do about that?"

If the person with cancer must take other pills, then never give them on an empty stomach unless the label instructs you to do so. Otherwise, offer Maalox, dry bread, or saltine crackers beforehand, or give the medicine after a meal.

If the person with nausea is taking potassium pills or potassium liquid, talk with the pharmacist or nurse about its side effects. Potassium can cause nausea, which can make the nausea from chemotherapy worse. Ask the doctor about different ways to take potassium that may not cause so much nausea.

Think of other obstacles that could interfere with carrying out your plan

What additional roadblocks could get in the way of doing the things recommended in this chapter? For example, will the person with cancer cooperate? Will other people help? How will you explain your needs to other people? Do you have the time and energy to carry out the plan?

Develop plans for getting around these roadblocks using the six problem-solving steps discussed in the first section of this book (see pages xi–xvi).

Carrying Out and Adjusting Your Plan

Checking on results

You can check on how well your plan is working by keeping track of the number of times the person with cancer vomited, by asking how severe the feelings of nausea are, and by noticing how much he or she has cut back on normal activities because of nausea. You can use the chart below to help keep track.

Table 6. Nausea and Vomiting Chart

Day of Week	Number of times vomited	Severity of nausea (rate 0-10)	Amount of interference with activities (rate 0-10)
Monday			
Tuesday			
Wednesday			
Thursday			
Friday			
Saturday			
Sunday			

Rate severity: 0 = not at all; 5 = moderate; 10 = very severe
Rate amount of interference: 0 = did not cut back at all; 5 = cut back moderately; 10 = cut back all activities

If your plan doesn't work...

If problems with nausea are getting worse, review the list under *When to Get Professional Help* (pages 203–205). Ask yourself if you are doing everything you can to reduce this symptom. If the person is becoming anxious about getting nauseated or if the nausea is harder and harder to control, ask the doctor about other antinausea medicines or about reducing the chemotherapy dose.

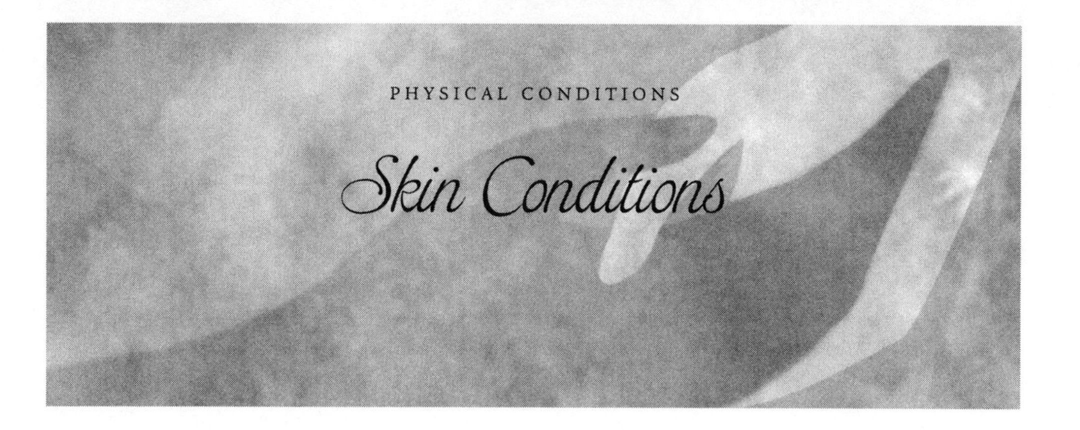

Skin Conditions

Understanding the Condition

Skin problems are not usually an emergency but can be upsetting and uncomfortable for the person who has them and can indicate other medical problems. As a family caregiver, you can help by noticing early signs of skin problems, by helping to treat them, and by encouraging the person with cancer to care for his or her skin.

Many people experience changes in their skin during cancer treatments. Sometimes chemotherapy causes skin changes. Some of these are more bothersome than others. The skin can become dry and itchy. Rashes or little sores can appear. Some people sweat more when receiving chemotherapy. Skin, veins, and fingernails may become darker. Chemotherapy may also make the person with cancer more prone to sunburn.

Radiation therapy causes skin problems that can last several weeks after treatments are completed. Typical skin reactions include dryness, itching, and redness. These reactions are confined to the areas where the radiation beam enters or exits the body. Radiation therapy to a warm, moist area, for example, the groin or armpit, is more likely to affect the skin than treatment to a dry area. Most of these reactions go away a few weeks after treatment is finished, but sometimes the treated skin stays dark long after treatment is over.

Some of these skin problems can be eliminated, some can be reduced, and some will not get better until treatments are completed. Almost all skin problems improve after treatments are over.

Your goals are to:

- call for professional help when it is needed
- relieve itching
- prevent dryness
- help conceal dark skin, veins, or nails

- treat acne
- limit sweating
- limit sun exposure
- take care of skin during and after radiation therapy

When to Get Professional Help

Call the doctor or nurse if any of the following conditions exist:

- ▲ **Skin gets very rough, red, or painful.** If you see these skin changes, report them. Also report any new drugs or lotions that are being used. Roughness or redness may signal an allergic skin reaction to a new medicine. If chemotherapy was started recently, if the dose was changed, or if new drugs were added to the chemotherapy list, report these changes, too. The cause of redness or roughness may also be external, for example, an allergic reaction to a detergent or soap or new food. Therefore, also report any new lotions or soaps the person with cancer is using or new foods he or she is eating.
- ▲ **A cut becomes very red, sore, or swollen.** Report any cuts that are not healing. They may become painful when lightly touched, and the skin around the cut may become shiny, red, and raised. If you act early, you can prevent serious skin infections.
- ▲ **Pus comes out of an opening or cut.** Pus usually indicates a skin infection. Pus from any opening should be reported.
- ▲ **A rash or hives starts.** These conditions could be caused by a drug reaction, a reaction to food or liquid, or too tight clothing over a dressing. If you do not know what caused this skin problem and the person with cancer has no history of rashes or hives, then it's best to call.
- ▲ **Severe itching lasts more than three days.** Itching can be a very bothersome side effect of a drug. It can also be caused by the release of chemicals through the skin that the body cannot process–the excess substances get pushed through the pores of the skin.
- ▲ **Skin is scratched open and looks red.** If itching becomes severe, the person may scratch the skin open and not even realize it. Red and open skin can become infected.

- ▲ **Skin turns yellow.** Color changes on the skin signal a major organ is not working well. For example, if a person turns yellow, this can mean the liver is not working correctly.
- ▲ **A bruise does not improve in a week.** Bruises that do not heal can mean the platelet counts are low, and very slow bleeding may still be occurring at the site of the bruise.

Know the answers to the following questions before you call the doctor or nurse:

This information will help the doctor or nurse determine the seriousness of the reported skin problems and what to do about them.

- When did the problem start? ____________________
- What do you think brought it on? ____________________
- How bad or embarrassing is it to the person? ____________________
- What helps it feel or look better? ____________________
- What is the person's temperature? ____________________
- How long does it take a bruise to go away? ____________________
- If there is a rash, what makes it appear and when does it go away? ____________________
- Are there any cuts that are not healing? ____________________
- If there is itching, where is it and what relieves it? ____________________
- When was the last chemotherapy treatment? ____________________
- What other medicines are being taken and at what doses? ____________________
- When was the last radiation treatment and to what area of the body? ____________________

If a new chemotherapy regimen has been started recently, report this along with the skin problems. Hives or a red rash that is bothersome or itches suggests an allergic reaction. If chemotherapy was started recently, if the dose was changed, or if new drugs were added to the chemotherapy list, report these medication changes. Red, rough, or painful skin usually signals an unusual reaction to a medication.

Here is an example of what you might say when calling:

"My wife is Dr. Testa's patient. She scratched her skin open. She's been itching for days, and now the skin on her arm has broken open."

What You Can Do to Help

Here are some things you can do to deal with skin problems:

- relieve itching
- prevent dryness and itching
- help conceal dark skin, veins, or nails
- treat acne
- limit sweating
- limit sun exposure
- help care for skin during and after radiation therapy

Relieve itching

The following is a list of things you can do to help relieve itching:

Suggest bathing with cool water and using gentle soap. Hot water can damage and dry out skin tissues. Harsh soaps are also too drying and should be avoided. Try an oatmeal soap or one with oil—be careful because they can make the tub slippery. Alpha Keri may be added to bath water. It eliminates the need for soap and softens the skin.

Add baking soda to bath water. Baking soda soothes sensitive skin and decreases itching.

Remind the person with cancer to rinse skin thoroughly and pat dry.

Suggest using skin lotions to help keep skin moist.

Apply cool, moist compresses to itchy areas. Cool soaks are soothing and relieve itching at least for a short time. Use washcloths or soft dish towels soaked in cool water and wrung out.

Suggest keeping nails short and clean. Shorter, well-filed nails are less likely to scratch open the skin.

Encourage wearing clean white gloves, if scratching. Clean white gloves over the hands help prevent scratching the skin with the nails. They are especially helpful at night when the person does not know he or she is scratching.

Change bed sheets daily. Dry skin flakes off and gathers on bed sheets. This can cause more itchiness and can further dry out the skin. Changing the sheets frequently removes the dry skin flakes and helps eliminate a buildup of bacteria. Fresh sheets bring a sense of comfort as well.

Wash sheets and towels in gentle laundry soap, such as Dreft or Ivory Snow. Harsh detergents remain on clothes, towels, and sheets and can cause itching and irritation.

Avoid harsh laundry detergents. Detergents that attack oil or stains have more chemicals that are irritating to tender skin. Gentle detergents are made for softer, tender skin and should be used if skin problems occur.

Keep the room cool at 60° to 70°F. When the body sweats more, itchiness increases.

Encourage rest. Too much activity makes the skin sweat. Rest cools the skin down again and decreases itchiness or skin irritation.

Avoid extreme cold or heat.

Suggest covering up in the sun. Heat from the sun causes sweating. Covering up also prevents sunburn and drying out of the skin. Use a lotion with at least an SPF 15 sunblock.

Prevent dryness and itching

Dryness leads to itching. Both can break the skin tissues to the point of cracking open. Here are a number of things you can encourage the person with cancer to do to prevent or treat dry skin:

Add mineral oil or baby oil to bath water. The oil soaks in and prevents the water from drying out the skin. However, be careful since it could make the tub slippery. Put a rubber mat in the tub to prevent falls.

Encourage taking sponge baths instead of full baths or showers. They are cooler and decrease the amount of time the skin is immersed in water.

Use premoistened towelettes. A new product available is a packet of premoistened towelettes that can be placed in the microwave. These towelettes contain a cleansing/moisturizing liquid that does not need to be rinsed off.

Use warm, not hot water. Hot showers and tub baths expose more skin to drying heat.

Do not scrub the skin. Scrubbing pulls on delicate skin tissues and removes important moisture.

Pat skin dry. Patting is more gentle than rubbing and helps lock in needed moisture.

Suggest applying a mild, water-based moisturizing cream to skin when it is still slightly moist after a bath. Water-based lotions replace needed moisture. Alcohol-based lotions dry out the skin and should be avoided.

Limit bathing to once a day or less. Bathing more than once a day leads to excessive dryness because the skin is rubbed and exposed to soap and hot water.

Encourage drinking two quarts (eight glasses) of fluid every day, unless otherwise instructed. Drinking fluids reduces the risk of dehydration and restores moisture to skin tissues.

Avoid extreme heat, cold, or wind. Heat, cold, and wind chafe the skin, damaging it as well as drying it out.

Avoid colognes, after-shaves, or after-bath splashes that contain alcohol. These dry the skin.

Remind the person with cancer to use an electric razor. Electric razors are less likely than razor blades to scrape off layers of skin.

Avoid opening or popping blisters, and put dry clean gauze on any open areas.

Help conceal dark skin, veins, or discolored fingernails

Skin pigment is affected by chemotherapy and often turns darker. If this is bothersome to the person with cancer, suggest the following:

Wear long sleeves to hide dark veins. They also provide some protection against bumping or bruising.

Women may wish to apply a thin layer of make-up foundation on their skin.

Keep nails clean, short, and filed smoothly. Women may want to wear nail polish.

Treat acne

Changes in skin pores and skin discharges can lead to blemishes that are both uncomfortable and unsightly. Here are some things you can encourage the person with cancer to do to prevent or treat acne:

Keep skin clean with mild soap and warm water. Harsh soaps inflame blemishes and strip the skin of important moisture.

Pat skin dry. Gentle drying allows new skin to heal and doesn't irritate reddened or swollen areas.

Avoid astringents. Although they dry out blemishes, astringents also dry the whole face and remove too much moisture. Keeping the skin clean is the best treatment for acne caused by chemotherapy.

Limit sweating

Encourage the person with cancer to dress in two light layers of clothing. Chemotherapy can cause excessive amounts of perspiration. The layer closest to the body should be cotton to absorb moisture. The outer layer should be light to allow air to pass through.

Change damp or wet clothing or bed sheets as soon as possible. Damp or wet cloth locks in sweat, which can lead to chills and discomfort.

Limit sun exposure

Chemotherapy makes the skin tissue especially sensitive to the sun's rays, and sunburn occurs rapidly. Encourage the person receiving chemotherapy to do the following:

Cover legs and arms. Clothing stops the sun's rays from damaging the skin.

Wear lightweight fabrics. They allow more air to pass through to the skin and keep it dry. Covering also protects the skin from the sun's rays.

Wear a wide-brimmed hat and sunglasses.

Use a suntan lotion with a sunblock of SPF 15 or higher. It prevents harmful rays from burning the skin. Remind the person to reapply sunblock at least every hour if hot and sweaty. Sunburn can occur in as little as 15 minutes of direct sunlight. Also apply on overcast days because ultraviolet rays can penetrate the clouds.

Apply sunscreen to any newly exposed scalp.

Stay in direct sun only for a short time.

Stay out of the sun from 10:00 A.M. to 4:00 P.M. The sun is hottest and most dangerous during these hours. The skin tissues are very sensitive to these rays while the person with cancer is receiving certain chemotherapy drugs. Ask the doctor or nurse about this. They'll tell you if the drugs cause extra sensitivity to the sun.

Take care of skin during and after radiation therapy

Encourage the person receiving radiation therapy to do the following:

Wash with lukewarm water and mild soap. Wash the skin gently and avoid very hot or cold water. Do not scrub the skin because this irritates it. Lukewarm water and gentle rinsing is best.

Keep the treatment area clean and dry. A daily sponge bath or lukewarm shower is recommended. If sweating occurs, cleanse afterwards.

Avoid using scented or medicated lotions, rubbing alcohol, creams, body oils, talcums, perfumes, and antiperspirants. All of these skin ointments irritate the skin. Many leave a coating on the skin that can interfere with radiation therapy or healing. A special cream may be allowed by the radiation therapy department. Staff will recommend it and explain how to use it.

Avoid cornstarch to control perspiration. Cornstarch will clump and cause a wet covering. Dusting with cornstarch or any talcum is to be avoided. Report wet skin areas to clinic staff, who will suggest how to treat them if they are near areas treated by radiation. Wet or moist areas are more likely to appear in skin folds, under the arms, and in the groin.

Avoid ice packs. Ice irritates the skin. It constricts the blood vessels, which may inhibit healing.

Avoid hot water bottles and heating pads. Heat can also irritate the skin.

Avoid direct sunlight to treated skin. The ultraviolet rays of the sun can burn the treated skin easily because the layer of skin where treated is very tender during and after radiation.

Wear loose clothing. Tight clothing causes redness and irritation. Loose clothing lets the skin breathe and does not restrict its flexibility.

Avoid scratching treated skin. Scratching, rubbing, or scrubbing must be avoided. This can cause infection, irritation, or soreness. If itchiness is a problem, consult with the doctor or nurse.

Possible Obstacles

Think about what could stop you from carrying out your plan and how you would deal with it.

Here are some obstacles that other people have faced:

"It's only the skin and not the body."

Skin problems need to be treated early to prevent infection and to decrease discomfort. If you notice changes, talk them over with the nurse or doctor. Don't wait until an infection or severe discomfort occurs.

"No one seems to know what to do about this itching. I guess we'll just have to live with it."

Itching is a difficult problem to heal. Try a combination of strategies to relieve constant itching. Keep experimenting and visit a dermatologist, if necessary.

"I'm afraid my skin will be fried by radiation therapy."

Radiation therapy does cause skin changes. The intention is not to "fry" the skin. Although it does get red and sensitive, the skin will heal. Be sure to call for help, especially if the skin gets moist or wet and becomes sore. Clinic staff keep a close watch on the skin, and the radiation therapist may postpone the treatment to give the skin a rest.

Think of other obstacles that could interfere with carrying out your plan

What additional roadblocks could get in the way of doing the things recommended in this chapter? For example, will the person with cancer cooperate? Will other people help? How will you explain your needs to medical staff? Do you have the time and energy to carry out the plan?

Develop plans for getting around these roadblocks using the six problem-solving steps discussed in the first section of this book (see pages xi–xvi).

Carrying Out and Adjusting Your Plan

Checking on results

Check the skin regularly to see if it has changed since radiation or chemotherapy began. Keep records of the skin problems the person with cancer is having and of what helps or makes them worse. These records will be helpful to health professionals in diagnosing and treating the problems.

If your plan doesn't work...

If skin problems are getting worse, or if the person with cancer is becoming more and more uncomfortable or upset about these problems, review the section on *What You Can Do to Help* (pages 214–219). If you have done all you can, then ask the nurse or doctor for help. Tell them what you have done and what the results have been.

Vein Conditions (Needle Sticks)

Understanding the Condition

Many chemotherapy treatments are injected into veins, and veins are used to obtain samples for blood and diagnostic tests. People may also become anxious about these "needle sticks." Family caregivers can be helpful by 1) encouraging the person receiving needle sticks to do things to make it easier, 2) helping the person relax and attend to other things before and during needle sticks, and 3) helping to prepare skin and veins for needle sticks, and limiting discomfort.

It is important to protect the veins of anyone receiving treatment for cancer. Some people have a difficult time having their blood drawn or having needles put into their veins because the veins become sore or are hard to find and use. This chapter explains what you can do to minimize these problems as well as some alternative ways to get blood or give drugs without needle sticks in the arms.

After treatments are over, most people's veins return to normal. In some cases, veins can be damaged for a long time. Chemotherapy sometimes causes sclerosis of the veins, which means they harden and cannot be punctured again.

Needle sticks are, for the most part, unavoidable. You need to help the person with cancer protect his or her veins and prevent undue anxiety about this procedure. You also need to learn about the different ways to draw blood or to give medicines into the veins since some may be less upsetting than others.

Your goals are to:

- call for professional help when it is needed
- prepare veins and skin for needle sticks
- limit discomfort or anxiety during needle sticks

- know about alternatives to needle sticks and the new ways to inject drugs and draw blood
- learn how to care for IV tubes and feeding tubes, if used

When to Get Professional Help

The three symptoms listed below indicate a serious skin or vein problem. Each needs to be evaluated and treated by a health professional.

Call the doctor or nurse if any of the following conditions exist:

- ▲ **Aching, tenderness, swelling, or redness (particularly a red streak) anywhere on the arm where the needle stick (venipuncture) was done.** Report these problems so the nurse can decide whether the person needs to come into the clinic to have the arm or vein inspected. These symptoms might mean the skin or vein is reacting to the drug. The staff can also tell you over the telephone how to treat the problem, such as by putting ice on the skin or using warm compresses.
- ▲ **Any drainage, pus, or blisters at the site where a needle stick was done.** Clear or yellow-colored liquid coming from the needle stick site could mean an infection. Blisters also have fluid in them and should be reported.
- ▲ **The person is so upset or nervous about needle sticks he or she is considering skipping the treatment or procedure.** A few people become so anxious about having their blood drawn it stops them from going to a clinic appointment, visiting the lab, or having blood drawn. Professional staff know how to help. Address this problem early before it interferes with treatment.

Know the following information before you call:

- When did the skin or vein problem start? ___________________
- Where are the veins that are sore? ___________________________

- When was chemotherapy given or a blood draw done that made the sites sore? What chemotherapy was given? ______________

  ____

- Is there a dark black or blue bruise or any red streaks? ________

Here is an example of what you might say when calling:

"My father is Dr. Eisler's patient. His skin is swollen at the injection site. Chemotherapy was given yesterday at 2:00 P.M., and he noticed the swelling when we got home."

What You Can Do to Help

If the problem is not an emergency, there are some things you can do to help with sore veins and needle sticks:

- prepare the skin and veins for needle sticks
- limit discomfort and anxiety during needle sticks
- learn about alternatives to needle sticks into arm veins
- learn how to care for IV tubes and feeding tubes, if used

Prepare the skin and veins for needle sticks

Encourage staying warm. Warmth makes the veins relax and fill up with blood. Sometimes the chemotherapy nurses wrap the arm in a warm, wet cloth a few minutes before an injection. This helps the veins to be easily seen.

Encourage eating well the day before the treatment. Food and fluids help maintain good blood flow through the veins. On the day of treatment, the person with cancer should eat and drink normally in the morning unless he or she is scheduled for tests that require fasting (going without solid foods for a period of time).

Encourage drinking two to three quarts (eight to ten glasses) of liquid every day, if possible. Fluids dilate or inflate the veins. Blood flows better and the veins are more likely to stick up and be found easily. Encourage the person with cancer to drink as much as possible, unless fluids are restricted for other reasons, such as heart disease.

Encourage taking a walk while waiting for chemotherapy or a blood draw. Walking to the clinic or near the clinic area helps increase good blood flow and keeps the veins pumped up.

Encourage exercising the hands and arms at home. Exercising at home can help veins inflate. Encourage the person with cancer to squeeze a rubber ball or lift small weights, like cans of soup. He or she can do this while talking with family or friends or watching television.

Encourage using moisturizer lotions. Apply a favorite lotion, cream, or ointment to the skin from fingertips to elbows. Lotion keeps the skin moisturized, which prevents dryness, cracking, and thickening of the skin. When the skin is dry, it's harder and more painful to puncture with a needle. The best time to apply moisturizers is after the skin has been wet—after bathing, showering, swimming, or doing dishes. Pat the skin almost dry and then apply the lotion. Do this as often as possible, at least four times each day.

Limit discomfort and anxiety during needle sticks

Needle sticks make many people anxious. There are several things you can do to help reduce or minimize any anxiety:

Give antinausea medicines, which also promote relaxation. Check with the doctor or nurse about giving antinausea medicines before chemotherapy treatments. Many of these medicines also decrease anxiety.

Talk about pleasant experiences while waiting. Have the person with cancer talk and think about pleasant experiences while waiting for treatment or a blood draw.

Suggest doing an activity to take the mind off the treatments. Reading an interesting magazine or talking with another person in the waiting room about something pleasant can help. Bring a portable cassette or CD player to listen to music or relaxation tapes.

Remind the person to look away from the arm. Many lab workers and nurses distract the person receiving a needle stick by talking with them. Suggest the person also look somewhere else in the room during the procedure.

Talk to the doctor and nurse about the anxiety. The doctor may prescribe a medicine to make the person more relaxed or may recommend a mental health professional to help with these feelings.

Encourage practicing deep breathing and other relaxation techniques and use these skills when receiving IV treatments or needle sticks. Relaxation is a skill and improves with practice. When the person with cancer practices at home, he or she can then use that skill to relax in medical settings.

Ask about the use of products that numb the skin, such as EMLA cream, if the person with cancer finds needle sticking very painful.

Learn about alternatives to needle sticks into arm veins

If needle sticks are a continuing problem or if the person with cancer is going to be receiving many of them over time, there are other ways to get blood out of the body for routine tests and other ways to get drugs into the body. Three options are available at most large medical centers and have been used by many people with cancer for the last 10 to 20 years.

1. *Ask about finger sticks for some blood draws.* Sometimes a finger stick–a pin prick on the finger that gives only a drop or two of blood–is all that is needed for certain tests, such as a complete blood count (CBC) or platelet count. Ask your nurse or lab technician if this is an option for some tests.

2. *Ask about IV catheters that connect to large veins.* These catheters are special small, flexible, and sterile tubes that can be put into large blood vessels under the skin. They are the same size as most IV lines. They can stay in for months and are taped to the chest or arm. These catheters, sometimes called Broviacs, Hickmans, or PICC lines, are used to draw blood for lab tests and to inject medicine or drugs used in chemotherapy into a large vein. Some people choose to have these inserted to avoid needle sticks in the arms and hands. If the person with cancer is interested in finding out more about these options, ask the nurse or doctor.

3. *Ask about permanent ports or access devices that can be placed under the skin.* Another way to get drugs into the body without sticking a vein every time is through a permanent port site. These are small (about one inch), metal discs that are placed under the skin, usually

on the chest. A small IV line extends from them into a large vein. If you press lightly on the skin, you can feel them, but they are barely visible from the outside.

If an IV catheter or a permanent port are being considered, here are some questions that will help determine which of the two is better for the person with cancer:

- How often does the catheter or port need to be flushed to stay open, and who will do this?

  Ports need to be flushed only once every four weeks if no drugs are given and no blood is taken. The person with cancer can visit a doctor's office or clinic and have this done. Visiting nurses can also do this at home if it is too hard for the person with cancer to travel. Some people with cancer or caregivers learn to do this themselves, but it takes good control of the fingers and good vision to do it alone.

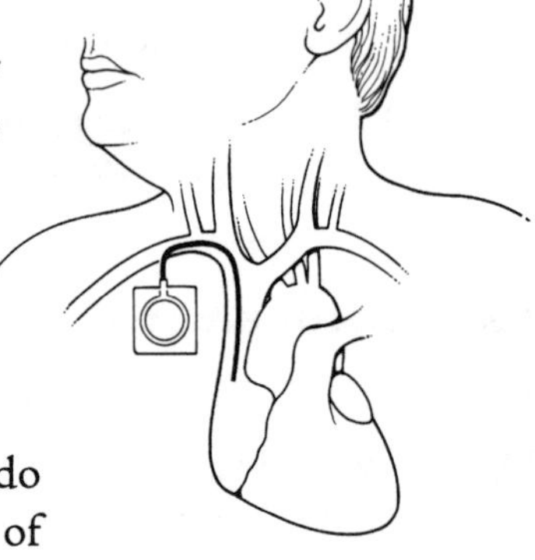

Permanent port

  Intravenous catheters in the chest must be flushed every day to keep them open and available for future use. However, the dressing around them needs to be changed only three times per week. Again, caregivers and family members can learn to do this at home.

- How much can a person move and exercise with catheters and ports?

  Ports do not prevent athletic exercise. Because the port is under the skin, the person with cancer can swim, play sports, and do any athletic activity he or she wants.

  Catheters hang outside of the body, so swimming and some athletic sports are not advised because the catheter might be pulled out.

- Will the treatments he or she receives be better with catheters or with ports?

  Some medical centers require a catheter be used with certain drugs. People with leukemia, for example, need to have a catheter inserted to receive large amounts of IV fluids and drugs. Ask which method the medical center prefers to use, and use the one they recommend.

Learn how to care for IV tubes and feeding tubes, if used

If the person you are caring for has IV or feeding tubes when at home, you will have to learn how to manage their care. Nurses can show you how to care for the skin around the tubes and how to mix and give medicines or food through the tubes, if ordered by the doctor. If you have problems, you can ask for a nurse to visit your home to help you solve problems.

Possible Obstacles

Think about what could prevent you from managing problems with veins.

Here are some obstacles other caregivers have faced:

"The staff didn't say anything about ports or catheters, so I assumed that they shouldn't be used."

The staff may not know how upsetting needle sticks are to the person with cancer, so they may not think it is a problem. If it takes three or more attempts to do needle sticks in the arms, ask about the availability and advisability of using ports or catheters.

"I've had trouble with needle sticks all my life, so nothing can be done."

Health care staff who give cancer treatments are usually very experienced doing needle sticks. They have had special training in how to do this procedure, and they understand how difficult this can be for some people. Therefore, you may find needle sticks in a cancer clinic are much less of a problem than you thought they might be.

Think of other obstacles that could interfere with carrying out your plan

What additional roadblocks could get in the way of doing the things recommended in this chapter? For example, will the person with cancer cooperate? Will other people help? How will you explain your needs to medical staff? Do you have the time and energy to carry out the plan?

Develop plans for getting around these roadblocks using the six problem-solving steps discussed in the first section of this book (see pages xi–xvi).

Carrying Out and Adjusting Your Plan

Checking on results

- Are nurses and laboratory technicians able to find veins during needle sticks?
- Is the skin near the veins moist and unbruised?
- Is the person with cancer worried or upset about needle sticks?
- If there are problems with needle sticks, have alternative ways of drawing blood or giving medicines been considered?

If your plan doesn't work...

If problems with veins are getting worse, or if the person with cancer is becoming more and more anxious, review this chapter. If you have done all you can, then ask the nurse or doctor about the different options for IV lines or ports on a short- or long-term basis.

Living with Cancer and Cancer Treatments

This section provides information about living with cancer after treatment. The chapters include *Hair Loss, Lymphedema, Mobility (Moving Around the House), Ostomies and Prostheses, Sexual Conditions,* and *Tiredness and Fatigue.*

The information in this section fits most situations, but yours may be different. If the doctor or nurse tells you to do something else, follow what they say. If you think there may be a medical emergency, see the *When to Get Professional Help* section of each chapter.

This section explains conditions that many people with cancer face. Encourage the person with cancer to read this information, and then you can work together as a team.

Hair Loss

Understanding the Condition

Hair loss can be very upsetting to many people receiving treatments for cancer. It is a highly visible reminder to them and others of their illness. As a family caregiver, you can help by encouraging the person with cancer to prepare for hair loss before it happens. Knowing what to expect and being prepared for what happens can greatly reduce the stress and social isolation that can occur.

Some chemotherapy treatments can cause partial or complete hair loss. This may start as early as 7 to 14 days after treatment begins, and hair may not grow back until 6 to 12 months after chemotherapy treatments are completed. Radiation to the head may cause permanent hair loss. Depending on where the radiation is directed, hair can also be lost on the eyelashes, eyebrows, pubic area, arms, underarms, chest, and legs.

When hair does grow back it may be different in texture. New hair may also be a different color because of a temporary absence of pigment in the hair shaft. If hair was brown, it might be lighter. Changes in color and texture are usually not permanent.

Ask the physician, nurse, or technician what to expect about hair loss with the treatments the person with cancer is receiving.

- When will the hair loss start?
- Will it fall out suddenly or slowly?
- How much of the hair will be lost?
- When will it grow back?

Your goals are to:

- help the person with cancer care for the scalp and get a wig or head cover
- help them cope during the time the hair is missing

When to Get Professional Help

Call the doctor or nurse if the hair loss is unexpected or gets worse. You can also talk to a social worker or other mental health professional if the person with cancer feels extremely distressed about the hair loss or is having difficulty adjusting.

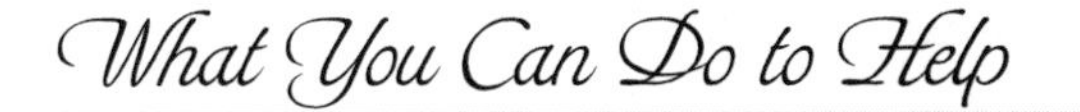

There are some things you can do to help the person with cancer deal with hair loss:

- care for the scalp and help them cope
- get a wig or head cover

Caring for the scalp and coping with hair loss

Encourage the person losing hair to do the following:

Consider getting a shorter hair style before treatments begin. The person with cancer will have time to adjust to a new look.

Gently brush and wash away hair that is falling out.

Gently clean hair and scalp with a mild protein shampoo twice a week. Use gentle shampoos for dry or damaged hair. Also massage the scalp to remove skin scales.

Gently wash off loose hair from other parts of the body using a mild soap.

Use a satin pillow or hair net while sleeping. A satin pillow prevents tangling, and hair sheds more evenly when held in a net.

Consider cutting or shaving the last few remaining hairs. When almost all hair is gone, the last strands can tickle or irritate the scalp leading to scratching.

AS HAIR GROWS BACK

Use a protein conditioner. Conditioners add body to fine or limp hair. It takes time for new hair shafts to become thick.

Avoid hair care products that contain bleach, peroxide, ammonia, alcohol, or lacquer. Avoid hair dyes and products with harsh chemicals.

Select hairstyling products such as mousses, sprays, or gels that have light or normal hold. These can be shampooed out. Stronger products build up on hair shafts and can damage remaining hair or new hair.

Avoid heat, curling irons, hot rollers, or blow dryers as much as possible. Gently towel dry hair or use a blow dryer set at the lowest setting. Keep heat farther away from the scalp than usual because the skin is sensitive and may easily burn.

Avoid braids or ponytails, and use a wide-toothed comb. Pulling breaks very fragile hair. Comb it gently with a wide-toothed comb.

Postpone a perm on new hair. After chemotherapy, let new hair grow in and wait until the hair is at least three inches long to get a very mild body wave that lasts for a short time. Permanent waves cannot be tolerated by the scalp until at least nine months after chemotherapy.

Keep hair short and easy to style. New hair breaks easily. Long hair requires more curling, pinning, and combing than short hair. Shorter hairstyles are easier to maintain.

DURING TREATMENT ALWAYS

Protect the head and newly exposed skin from the sun with a hat and sunblock of SPF 15 or higher. Sun rays also dry the scalp and can burn it more readily than usual.

Wear a hat or a head scarf to retain heat in cold weather. Because heat is lost through the top of the head, wearing a hat or scarf retains body heat and protects the scalp from drying out in colder, harsh weather.

Wear sunglasses to protect the eyelashes. Even eyelashes are sensitive to chemotherapy and can be easily broken. Protection from the sun and cold weather is recommended.

Getting a wig or head cover

Encourage the person losing hair to do the following:

Ask a hairstylist about buying a wig. Hairstylists can call a wig supplier and order catalogs. They can describe the different kinds of wigs to the person with cancer and order the wig. Do this before all the hair is lost.

Call a wig shop in the phone book, and talk with professionals early about wigs. If you plan to buy a wig, be prepared to pay $30 or more. Some wigs cost as much as $100. Major department stores often carry wigs as well. Many people prefer to have their hairstylist order and style a wig specifically for them.

Match a small lock of the person's hair with a wig color before starting chemotherapy. Wigs come in many colors and textures. A hair stylist can make a close match to the person's hair color and style by seeing the person before the hair falls out and by having a lock of the person's hair.

Practice wearing the wig at home. The person will be more comfortable in public after wearing the wig at home and becoming used to it.

Try turbans, scarves, hats, or caps. Many stores sell attractive terry cloth or cotton turbans. Some hospital gift shops also carry these. Head coverings protect against drafts, enhance appearance, and retain body heat.

Talk with other people who have lost their hair because of cancer treatments. Different people cope differently with this problem. Some accept baldness and do not cover their heads except in cold weather. Others feel wigs or turbans are important and helpful. Getting their ideas helps the person with cancer judge what might be best for him or her.

Possible Obstacles

Here are some obstacles other people have faced in coping with hair loss:

"I can't afford a wig."

Some insurance companies (basic coverage or major medical) cover part or all of the cost of wigs because it is needed after a medical problem and is not for purely cosmetic reasons. To get insurance coverage, you might need a prescription, so check with your doctor.

"People say that he'll just have to live with being bald or having patches of hair on his head."

Appearance can be very important to the person with cancer. Losing one's hair can be quite upsetting. Helping a person look their best during a difficult time in their life can boost spirits and give confidence.

Think of other obstacles that could interfere with carrying out your plan

What additional roadblocks could get in the way of doing the things recommended in this chapter? For example, will the person with cancer cooperate? Will other people help? How will you explain your needs to medical staff? Do you have the time and energy to carry out the plan?

Develop plans for getting around these roadblocks using the six problem-solving steps discussed in the first section of this book (see pages xi–xvi).

Carrying Out and Adjusting Your Plan

Carrying out your plan

If possible, decide in advance whether the person with cancer wants a wig and what kind of a wig he or she wants. Order it as soon as possible.

If your plan doesn't work...

If your plan does not seem to be working or hair loss is getting worse and the person with cancer feels badly about it, ask the social worker, nurse, or hairstylist for help. Tell them what you have done and what the results have been.

LIVING WITH CANCER AND CANCER TREATMENTS

Lymphedema

Understanding the Condition

Lymphedema is the swelling of any limb (hand, wrist, arm, ankle, calf, or leg) due to insufficient drainage of the lymphatic system. It is caused by removal of lymph nodes during surgery or by radiation treatment that may damage or cause swelling in lymph nodes. Lymphedema is most common among women who have been treated for breast cancer and who may experience swelling of the arms or hands, but it can also occur among men treated for prostate cancer and people treated for abdominal or pelvic tumors who may experience swollen ankles or legs.

The lymphatic system is a network of thin vessels, lymph nodes (also called glands), and lymph fluid. It helps fight infection by circulating and filtering lymph, a clear liquid that carries immune cells throughout the body. The lymph fluid comes from the blood and returns to the blood through the lymph vessels. When the lymph system is damaged, the fluid does not drain properly and builds up in the limbs, making them swell. If untreated, the collection of fluid slows the healing of wounds and invites bacteria to grow, which can lead to infections. Lymphedema can also be quite uncomfortable and can make the limb feel heavy.

The onset of lymphedema is often subtle and unpredictable. There is no way of predicting who will or will not develop lymphedema. It can occur immediately after treatment or months or even years later. The potential for developing lymphedema continues throughout the person's lifetime, and when it does occur, lymphedema can have a profound effect on the person's quality of life.

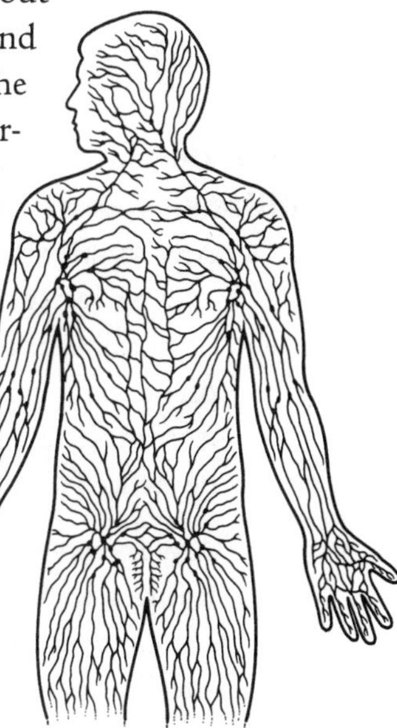

Lymphatic system

With proper education and care, many people can avoid lymphedema or, if it develops, keep it under control.

Sometimes an infection is the source of the problem, and this can be treated by antibiotics. If there is no infection, or the swelling continues after antibiotic therapy, a physical therapist should be consulted to develop a treatment plan. Treatment methods include:

- a compression sleeve that helps push fluids out of the swollen area
- manual lymphatic drainage (performed by a trained therapist), involves gentle massage to direct and stimulate lymphatic drainage
- use of a sequential gradient pump that reduces swelling by applying pressure to the limb in timed cycles

Your goals are to:

- call for professional help if it is needed
- help reduce the swelling
- help avoid infection, burns, and muscle strain in the limb with lymphedema

When to Get Professional Help

Call the doctor or nurse during office hours if any of the following conditions occur with the person with lymphedema:

- ▲ **Any swelling, tightness, redness, or signs of infection on the arm or leg that is affected by lymphedema.** These are all signs of possible infection on or under the skin. The limb with lymphedema can become infected more easily than other limbs, and it is important to report an infection in the early stages so it can be treated.
- ▲ **Any injury to the arm or leg that is affected by lymphedema.** Injuries include punctures from pointed objects, sunburns, or cuts and scratches from pets, sharp objects, and knives. These should be reported to a doctor or nurse who can decide if an antibiotic is needed or tell you what to watch for if an infection has developed.

▲ **Pain or discomfort caused by swelling from lymphedema.** Pain or discomfort are signals of infection. If the swollen skin aches or is tender to the touch, there may be an infection. Pain may also signal an infection before you can see swelling. Another reason for pain is fluid backing up. This could be a signal of other problems, which the doctor should investigate.

Know the following facts before calling the doctor or nurse:

- What surgery or radiation treatments has the person with cancer had and where in the body?__________________________________
- What things were done in the past to manage the lymphedema and how successful were they?__________________________________
- What has been done to control lymphedema during this episode and what have been the results? __________________________________
- If the problem is an injury, when did the injury occur and what has been done? __________________________________

Here is an example of what you might say when calling about lymphedema:

"My wife is Dr. Toledo's patient. Her right arm, which is where she has had lymphedema in the past, is red and swollen and feels hot. What should I do?"

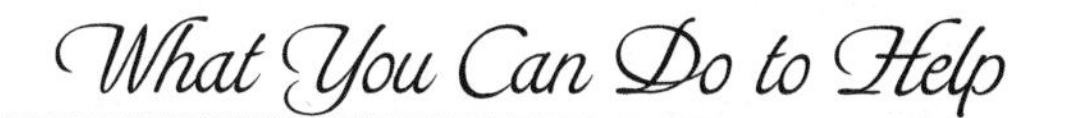

What You Can Do to Help

There are some things you can do at home to help the person with lymphedema:

- help reduce the swelling
- help avoid infections and muscle strain in the limb with lymphedema
- help avoid burns

Help reduce swelling

Encourage the person to elevate the arm or leg that is swollen. Prop up the arm or leg on a pillow. This will make it easier for fluid to drain from the swollen area.

Wrap the limb in an elastic ace wrap if the doctor or nurse has explained when and how to do this.

Encourage women with arm lymphedema to wear loose-fitting bras or breast prostheses. Avoid tight straps on the shoulders that can restrict circulation and make it harder for the lymph fluid to drain. Heavy prostheses pull on bra straps, which puts pressure under the arm and restricts fluid drainage.

Wear loose fitting clothing over the affected arm or leg. Avoid tight sleeves, socks, wristbands, and jewelry. Tight clothing can bind the skin and cut off circulation. It also restricts lymph and blood flow up the arm or leg.

Avoid using shoulder straps on suitcases, briefcases, purses, or bags if the person has arm lymphedema. Shoulder straps will cut into the skin, reduce circulation, and cause problems with lymph return.

Help avoid infections in the limb with lymphedema

Keep the limb with lymphedema clean and dry. Wash daily if the limb is sweaty or dirty. Dry the skin well after washing because damp skin lets bacteria grow.

Use moisturizing lotion. Dry skin gets infected more easily because bacteria enter through cracks in the skin. Lotion helps keep the skin flexible and prevents cracking.

Avoid using sharp objects. Be very careful using needles, pins, and knives. The skin will heal slowly, and infection may set in if punctured.

Use insect spray. Biting insects can pierce the skin and the skin will heal slowly if swollen from lymphedema. The bites can also cause infections.

Do not allow blood draws, needle injections, or blood pressure cuffs on the limb where lymph nodes have been removed or radiation was given. Punctures or pressure on the limb can cause swelling and infections. Tell technicians, nurses, and doctors about any lymphedema problems so that they can avoid hurting the affected area.

Clip and manicure nails carefully. Avoid tearing or cutting cuticles, which could cause infection. Instead, use a lanolin-based cream to soften cuticles.

Use an electric shaver to shave near a limb with lymphedema. For example, women with mastectomies should use an electric razor to shave under the arms. An electric razor is less likely than razor blades to damage the skin.

For arm or hand lymphedema, wear gloves when gardening. Hands are likely to be cut or punctured by thorns and sharp leaves or gardening tools when gardening.

For arm or hand lymphedema, wear rubber gloves when working with household cleaners, detergents, and bleaches. Household cleansers are very drying and can damage and crack the skin. Loose fitting gloves will protect the hands and will prevent skin damage from harsh chemicals.

Help avoid muscle strain in the limb with lymphedema

Encourage using the affected arm or leg as normally as possible. If the arm or leg with lymphedema is not used, muscles will become weak, and this may increase the likelihood of bruising or damaging the limb. Regular exercise may help keep the muscles toned.

Avoid heavy lifting. Heavy lifting will strain the limbs and pull muscles. Carry heavy packages or suitcases with the unaffected arm or side.

For arm or hand lymphedema, avoid scrubbing with the affected arm. Scrubbing, pushing, or pulling with the affected arm can make it swell more and damage muscles.

Help avoid burns

Encourage wearing protective clothing and sunscreen when in the sun. Use a sunscreen labeled SPF 15 or higher when in the sun. Avoid exposure to the sun between 10 a.m. and 3 p.m. This is when the sun is most likely to burn the skin.

Keep bath and dishwater lukewarm. Hot water can scald the skin. Scalded skin cracks and peels and is likely to become infected in a limb with lymphedema.

Use oven mitts and potholders. Oven mitts and potholders protect the skin from burning and scalding.

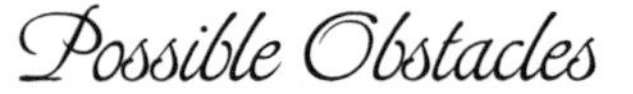

Here are some obstacles other people have faced in managing lymphedema at home:

"I forget to do everything I need to do to control my lymphedema."

Ask family members and friends to remind you and put a list of things to do someplace where you will see and notice it.

"I get so upset by my lymphedema that I don't want to think about it—and so I don't do some things I should to control it."

Try to separate, in your mind, the things you need to do from your lymphedema. Think of them as part of your normal routine. Also, ask family and friends to remind you about what to do without mentioning lymphedema.

Think of other obstacles that could interfere with carrying out your plan

What additional roadblocks could get in the way of doing the things recommended in this chapter? For example, will the person with cancer cooperate? Will other people help? How will you explain your needs to other people? Do you have the time and energy to carry out the plan?

Develop plans for getting around these roadblocks using the six problem-solving steps discussed in the first section of this book (see pages xi–xvi).

Carrying Out and Adjusting Your Plan

Checking on results

Controlling lymphedema takes time and patience. Look for small changes and improvements. Lymphedema problems will probably continue, but your goal is to help the person with cancer have an improved quality of life and for the episodes to be less severe.

If your plan doesn't work...

If lymphedema problems continue or if they are happening more often, encourage the person with lymphedema to talk to the doctor, and ask for a referral to a physical therapist if one has not been seen. Be sure the person with lymphedema is doing all the things listed in this chapter and recommended by the physician and physical therapist. If so, then keep doing them. Even if the problems continue, you are preventing the lymphedema from becoming worse.

LIVING WITH CANCER
AND CANCER TREATMENTS

Mobility (Moving Around the House)

Understanding the Condition

People with cancer can experience a variety of physical problems at different times during the course of treatment and over the length of illness. One problem that is particularly discouraging and potentially unsafe is when they have difficulty moving about, keeping balanced, bathing, or getting up from furniture because of feeling slowed down or weak.

Helping with transfers in the bathroom or around the home can be a challenge to many caregivers. If you have a bad back or health problems that prohibit lifting or straining, then helping the person with cancer may be especially difficult.

Many pieces of equipment make moving around, bathing, and transfers safer and easier for both of you. It's a matter of learning what is available and how to use the necessary equipment to the best advantage.

Your goals are to:

- call for help if there is an emergency
- increase the safety of the person with cancer during walking or moving
- locate and use equipment that helps with moving around in the home

When to Get Professional Help

Call the social worker or nurse if any of the following conditions exist:

- ▲ **You are not able to help the person move from one piece of furniture to another.**
- ▲ **You are not able to get the person from the house to the car.**
- ▲ **The person has fallen repeatedly or been hurt in a fall.**
- ▲ **The person with cancer needs oxygen all the time, and it is difficult for you to help him or her move around with the oxygen equipment.**

What You Can Do to Help

There are some things you can do on your own to help the person with cancer to move safely and comfortably:

- increase safety during walking or moving
- locate and use equipment that helps with moving around in the home

Increase safety during walking and moving

Inspect the bathroom and stairs for safety. Most accidents happen in these two places. Make sure objects on the floor are removed and railings are secure.

Install handrails in the shower or tub. Many people hang onto racks or shelves in the tub for steadiness. However, these can weaken and be pulled down. Handrails can be placed over the sides of tubs or installed directly into walls or shower stalls.

Place nonslip appliqués on the tub floor. These can be purchased at most pharmacies, supermarkets, or hardware stores and decrease chances of slipping while showering or getting in and out of a tub.

Remove loose rugs. Loose rugs are easy to slip on, especially when they are on linoleum and wooden floor surfaces.

Use a steady shower chair in the bathtub. Shower chairs make bathing or showering much safer. The larger the chair, the steadier it is. Some shower chairs even stretch over the side of the tub so a person can sit on the bench and slide over to the tub without too much lifting or shifting of body weight.

Install a showerhead with a flexible hose that can be held in the hand and directed to specific areas of the body.

Use wheelchairs or commodes with lift-off arms and lift-off footrests. When these chairs have a lift-off arms and footrests, they can be positioned alongside a bed or couch, and a person can lift the arm off and easily slide over to the new seat.

Raise beds, toilets, chairs, and couches to make it easier to move onto and off of them. If the height of a bed is low, getting out of it can be difficult. The bed can be raised on wooden blocks for a safer and easier transfer. Toilets are often too low, and a raised toilet seat can be purchased to elevate it anywhere from four to six inches. Chairs and couches can be dangerously low and lead to strains and even fractures when one is trying to rise out of them. Again, wooden blocks can be placed under furniture to raise it to safer heights.

Try sliding boards between seats to help with awkward transfers. Sliding boards are short pieces of wood that stretch between a wheelchair, for example, and a bed. The person does not have to stand to get from one place to another but shimmies across the board to the new setting.

Consider using Lifeline, a telephone service, to get help from neighbors. Lifeline is a button that is worn around the neck or placed near the person with cancer with which he or she can signal a neighbor for help. Most local community hospitals have this service. Look in the telephone book or call the hospital and ask for the Lifeline telephone number and contact person. Someone will interview you over the telephone and explain the monthly rental service. Sometimes financial discounts are available. You will need to name three neighbors who would agree to keep a key to the home and respond to a call from a central operator if the button is pushed. This system is an alternative to calling 911 or the emergency response unit.

Locate and use equipment that helps with moving around in the home

Ask if the hospital or home care agency has their own supply stores. Some have their own supply houses as well as personnel who will help you look at different options for home care.

Call a local medical equipment store to find out what they have to solve problems with moving. Most medical supply stores can advise you on the telephone about options in equipment for use at home. They know which kinds of equipment prescribed by a doctor are covered by insurance.

Pick up a home care catalog. Many pharmacies and some large department stores with catalog services have catalogs that picture and describe a variety of home care equipment and devices.

Ask service groups about donated equipment. Different service groups collect and repair equipment, such as wheelchairs and commodes. If a relative or friend belongs to a group that does this in your community, then ask them to approach the appropriate leaders, explain the need, and look over donated supplies.

Possible Obstacles

Here is an obstacle that others have had in solving problems with moving the person with cancer safely and comfortably:

"My father won't use the equipment I got to help him get around."

Discuss together what the problem is and what you will do to deal with it. If he does not agree there is a problem for him, then explain how it is a problem for you. Ask him to use the equipment for your sake. If he cannot understand your point of view, then get help from other people such as other family members, friends, or health professionals to help explain the problem to him.

If he does not want to have other people see him using the equipment, then put it away when there are guests. If he forgets to use the equipment, work out ways to remind him—for example, putting up signs—or he can practice using the equipment so it becomes a habit.

Think of other obstacles that could interfere with carrying out your plan

What additional roadblocks could get in the way of doing the things recommended in this chapter? For example, will the person with cancer cooperate? Will other people help? How will you explain your needs to other people? Do you have the time and energy to carry out the plan?

Develop plans for getting around these roadblocks using the six problem-solving steps discussed in the first section of this book (see pages xi–xvi).

Carrying Out and Adjusting Your Plan

Carrying out your plan

Develop your plan with the person you are caring for. Try simpler solutions first—things you can do together with what you have in your home. Talk with nurses, social workers, physical therapists, or occupational therapists and ask for their suggestions. Look into borrowing equipment. If it can't be borrowed, look into renting if the equipment is going to be needed for a short time. Purchasing equipment can save money if it is needed for a long time.

Checking on results

Keep track of the problems he or she has in walking and moving. If a problem happens occasionally and it is not dangerous, you may want to wait to see if it becomes more frequent. If a problem is potentially dangerous and you are worried, then develop your plan before the problem becomes serious.

If your plan doesn't work...

If your plan does not seem to be working or the problems in walking and moving are getting worse, review the list in the *When to Get Professional Help* section (page 243). If any of the conditions listed there exist, call the social worker or nurse immediately.

If problems with moving around the house continue, ask the social worker or nurse for help. Tell them what you have done and what the results have been.

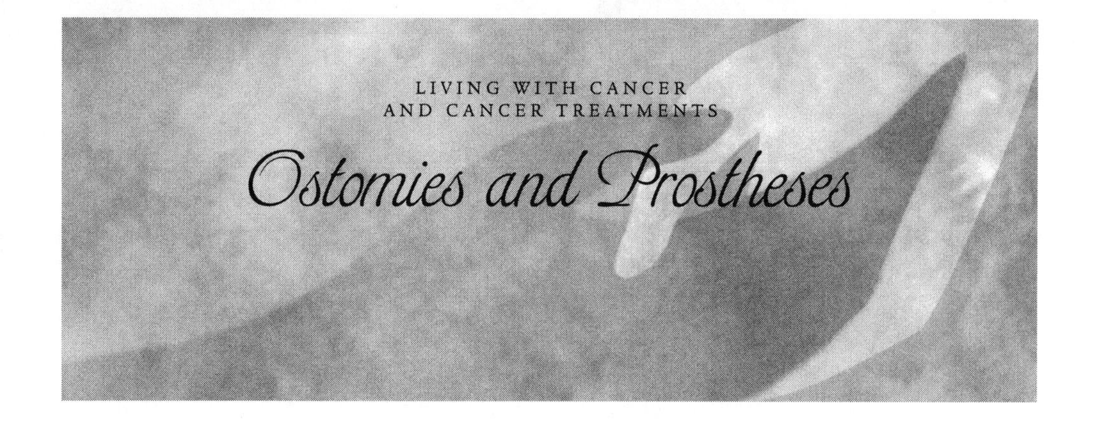

LIVING WITH CANCER
AND CANCER TREATMENTS

Ostomies and Prostheses

Understanding the Condition

An ostomy is a surgical opening. Prostheses are manmade substitutes for body parts that have been removed. Ostomies and prostheses are two different ways to help people return to a normal life after having organs removed by surgery. Both require learning to use the new body parts and sometimes an adjustment in lifestyle.

An ostomy is a surgically created opening that leads to the urinary or gastrointestinal canals or into the trachea (windpipe.) The whole connection—from the skin to the internal organ—is called an ostomy. The stoma is the part of an ostomy that you see on the skin. Ostomies are created to remove fluid or feces from the body or to allow air into the lungs.

Some ostomies are temporary so healing can take place. After healing, the ostomy is closed and the body resumes its normal function. Other ostomies are permanent. The person with cancer must learn how to care for the stoma—or the part of the ostomy that shows on the skin.

Prostheses replace body parts that have been removed. These body parts are often removed because they contain cancer that can spread. Examples of prostheses are breast, testicular, and leg prostheses and penile (penis) implants. Sometimes a prosthesis is put into the body during surgery such as a breast implant during breast reconstruction. Other times prostheses are placed in the body

Laryngectomy. Tissue removed.

long after surgery, such as a penile (penis) implant, which is placed 6 to 12 months after initial surgery. Other prostheses are external (outside the body). Examples of external prostheses are breast prostheses worn outside of the skin by women after a mastectomy or an artificial leg for someone who has had a leg amputation. All prostheses help people live independently and maintain their normal appearance. The cost of some prostheses are covered by health insurance with a prescription.

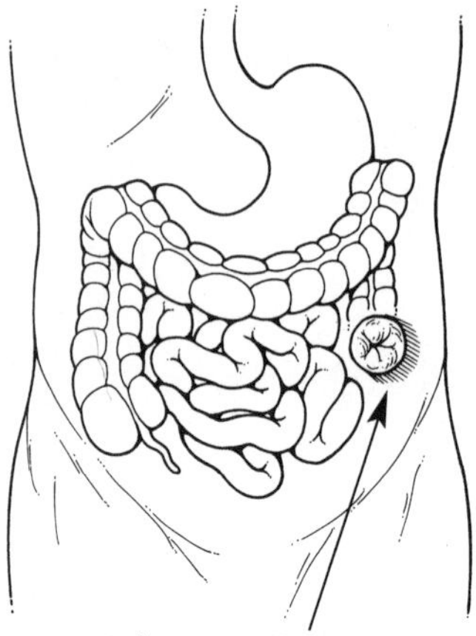

Colostomy. Stoma.

Your goals are to:

- know when to get professional help
- learn to care for an ostomy or stoma
- help the person with cancer select an external prostheses
- support the person with cancer in learning to cope with an ostomy or prosthesis

When to Get Professional Help

Call the doctor or nurse during office hours if any of the following conditions occur:

- **The person with cancer is having difficulty caring for an ostomy or stoma.** Health professionals such as respiratory therapists and nurses can teach the care of tracheal (windpipe) ostomies, and enterostomal therapists and nurses can teach the care of urinary or colon ostomies. They can visit the home if needed. Ask the doctor or nurse to arrange a teaching session.
- **The area around the stoma becomes red or swollen, is itchy, or develops bumps or a rash.** These symptoms could be caused by infection, by the pouch not fitting correctly, or they could be a skin reaction to the pouch or adhesive.
- **A prosthesis scrapes the skin or causes redness or pain.** This means the prosthesis is not fitted correctly and needs to be adjusted.

▲ **The person with cancer is confused about the type of prosthesis to purchase.** Talking with a doctor or nurse can help the person with cancer decide on a type of prosthesis that best meets his or her needs. They may refer the person with cancer to a specialist and may also tell about local support groups where people with the same conditions help each other.

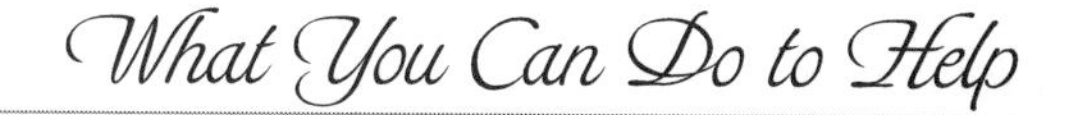

There are some things you can do at home to help the person with an ostomy or prosthesis:

- learn to care for an ostomy
- help decide about breast prostheses
- support the adjustment to leg, arm, or testicular prostheses

Learn to care for an ostomy

Assist with the care of tracheal ostomies following a total laryngectomy. Family caregivers should know how to care for a tracheal (windpipe) ostomy and be available to help the person with cancer when needed. You both should learn how to clean and care for the skin around the opening. You should also learn how to suction out mucous that can build up at the top of the windpipe. It is important to keep the air moist and humidified in the room to reduce problems with thick crusted mucous. You can help the person with cancer care for the ostomy and you can also remind him or her when care is needed.

Be available to assist with the care of urinary diversions. Urinary diversions drain urine out of the body through a stoma on the skin. Drainage is collected in small plastic pouches that are worn at all times. The skin care is important with an ostomy and skin must be thoroughly cleaned when the pouch is changed. You should know how to care for the ostomy and explain you are available to help if it is needed or wanted.

Be available to assist with the care of colostomies. A colostomy and an ileostomy are surgically created openings of the bowel. Many people wear a colostomy pouch over the stoma to collect the feces (bowel movement) that empties into the pouch. Others learn to regulate bowel movements so a pouch does not need to be worn at all times. Caring for the skin around the stoma and getting the right kind of pouch are challenges in the beginning. Sometimes the person with the colostomy is embarrassed to have help. If so, explain that you are available to help if it is needed or wanted.

Encourage the person with cancer to join a local ostomy club. In these groups, people with ostomies help each other by giving support and sharing experiences. Most large communities have ostomy clubs listed in the blue pages of the telephone book. They can also be found by calling the American Cancer Society or the social services department of your local hospital. Another group that can help you find a local club is the United Ostomy Association, Inc. (UOA) at (800) 826-0826 or www.uoa.org.

Help the woman with breast cancer decide about breast prostheses

Support her in deciding which type of external breast prosthesis is needed. Prostheses vary in type, weight, and color. Some replace an entire breast while others are small and worn by women after a lumpectomy or a segmental mastectomy. There are also nipple prostheses for when the nipple cannot be saved during breast reconstruction. Choosing a breast prosthesis is an important and personal decision. As a family caregiver, your support and encouragement can be very helpful—though it is important the woman make her own decision. One advantage of external prostheses is that they can be easily replaced if they are not satisfactory.

Call ahead to the medical supply store. External prostheses are sold in surgical supply stores and lingerie shops. Call to find out if they carry the type of prostheses desired and whether or not they have a professional fitter. Sometimes a custom-fitted one is needed.

Compare types of external breast prostheses and prices. Suppliers differ in the prices and the help they give. Shop around for the best fit and the right price. Using the telephone will save time and trips.

Encourage the person with breast cancer to wear a form-fitting top when shopping for a breast prosthesis. A form-fitting top will show the fit of a prostheses, which should be natural in contour and shape. A snugger top will also help the person with cancer see if the prosthesis stays in place when she moves.

Support the woman with breast cancer in deciding whether to have a breast implant. Breast implants are prostheses that are surgically inserted under the skin. They can be removed with surgery, but generally are left in for life. Some women prefer breast implants to an external breast prosthesis because their body looks more normal without clothes. They are also more convenient since there is no need to put on and take off the prosthesis every day. The decision to have breast implant is a very personal one and, as a caregiver, you can help by supporting whatever decision the woman with cancer makes. Since breast implants can be done at any time, there is no rush in making a decision. However, there are more options available if discussed at the time of diagnosis and treatment. She may want to experiment with an external breast prosthesis before deciding whether she wants an implant.

Support the adjustment to leg, arm, or testicular prostheses

Talk about the prostheses with the person with cancer, if desired. Sometimes people are hesitant to talk about getting a prosthesis. They may feel embarrassed or not want to upset others. You can help by expressing your willingness to talk about it—when he or she is ready and wants to. You can say you understand why the person feels hesitant but also explain that talking openly can help him or her think through the options and make a better decision.

Support the person with cancer while learning to use a new leg or arm prosthesis. Temporary leg or arm prostheses are usually fitted immediately after surgery to remove a limb. Permanent prostheses are fitted later after the wound has healed. In either case, it takes a while for a person to get used to using the new artificial limb. During this time emotional support from family caregivers is very helpful. You may also be able to help put on the prosthesis when he or she tries on a new limb and is learning to use it.

Support the decision to have or not have a testicular or penile implant. The decision to have or not have a testicular or penile implant is both personal and sensitive. Not all men feel they need or want an implant. However, for some, having the implant is very important. Both types of implants can be done at any time, and so there is no rush in making a decision. Whatever the man decides, he will appreciate your support of his decision.

Possible Obstacles

Think about what ideas or attitudes might prevent you from carrying out your plan and reaching the goal of assisting with the care of an ostomy or prostheses.

Here are some obstacles other people have faced:

"I could never learn to change this colostomy pouch."

"It does seem like a difficult thing to do, but I can help you learn to do it. Others have learned it. There are nurses and therapists who are specialists in this and who can teach us and even visit us at home if we need them."

"My husband won't let me help with his ostomy. He says it is too embarrassing. But he clearly needs help since he is having problems."

Nurses and therapists who specialize in ostomy care are skilled in dealing with feelings of embarrassment. Ask one of them for advice. It may be helpful for him to meet with the specialist who can explain that he does need help.

"My wife won't wear her prosthesis. She says it is uncomfortable, but she doesn't want to bother the doctor or nurse."

Her doctors and nurses want her to have the best care and this includes having the best prosthesis. Explain that they want her to tell them about her problems. If necessary, talk to the nurse yourself and she can encourage your wife to persist until she has a comfortable prosthesis.

Carrying Out and Adjusting Your Plan

Checking on results

It takes time to accept that an ostomy or prosthesis is a part of your life. Being patient and supportive is important. It also takes time to learn how to manage these new body parts. You should keep informed about what needs to be done and be available to help whenever the person asks. Your goal is to help make the ostomy or prosthesis a normal part of the person's life.

If your plan doesn't work...

If problems adjusting to the new body parts continue and don't seem to be getting better, encourage the person with cancer to talk to the doctor or nurse and to ask for a referral to a professional who specializes in helping people cope with ostomies or prostheses. If he or she remains very upset about the changes, suggest talking to a mental health professional. See the chapter *Depression* (pages 100–113) for more information on how to recognize severe emotional distress and what to do about it.

Sexual Conditions

Understanding the Condition

Sex is a very sensitive subject and coping with sexual problems requires careful thought and planning on the parts of both partners. Since sexual problems are rarely emergencies, there is time to plan and deal with the problems sensitively. The goal is for the person with cancer and his or her sexual partner to work together as a team.

Cancer and cancer treatments can affect a person's sexual desire, behavior, and pleasure, and adjusting to those changes is an important part of coping with the illness. It is important for the person with cancer and his or her partner to understand why sexual changes are happening, to know what to expect, and to know what they can do to deal with or adjust to those changes.

Sexual problems with cancer can have physical causes, emotional causes, or both. Physically, very few cancer treatments injure parts of the body that give orgasms or sexual enjoyment. Exceptions include treatments that affect the brain or spinal cord, certain surgeries such as mastectomy (removal of a breast) or orchiectomy (removal of testicles), drugs that change normal hormone balance, and radiation therapy to the lower abdominal and genital areas. Intercourse or sexual interactions may be impaired after these treatments, but people can still have feelings of pleasure. Side effects of treatments such as pain, nausea, or fatigue can also impair or reduce sexual pleasure. Finally, changes in the way a man or woman feels about their attractiveness can have an effect.

Adjusting to sexual changes due to cancer and cancer treatments

Talk over feelings or concerns. It is important for the person with cancer to discuss any fears or questions with his or her sexual partner. Talking about sexual matters with a close friend or medical professional can also help.

Plan periods of time for intimacy when you will not be interrupted. Privacy is important for relaxation and sexual pleasure. Planning for uninterrupted time might be difficult, but it will help the person with cancer and the partner give time and attention to intimacy that is needed.

A great deal of pleasure comes from touching and being held. Sexual intimacy can be achieved without intercourse, without orgasms, and without erections or ejaculations. Being held and touched is an important part of all sexual intimacy and may be even more important when other sexual activities are restricted. Intimacy can be expressed by holding hands, putting an arm around the waist or shoulders, rubbing the back or arms and legs, and any other type of touching. Touch brings comfort and security.

Your goals are to:

- know when professional help is needed
- understand the sexual effects of cancer and cancer treatments and what can be done to deal with these effects
- help the person with cancer prevent infections from sexual contact
- help the person with cancer experience sexual closeness and pleasure with his or her partner

When to Get Professional Help

Talk to the doctor or nurse if the person with cancer is experiencing any of the following:

- ▲ **Pain during intercourse.** Any pain with intercourse is a reason to talk to a doctor. Women should report painful intercourse to the gynecologist and ask for advice about trying other positions or about continuing intercourse. If a gynecologist has not been involved, report the pain to the surgeon or doctor in charge, who can make a referral to a gynecologist. Men should also report pain during intercourse and any redness on, or unusual discharge from, the penis. Radiation therapy to the abdominal or pelvic area may also cause pain during intercourse for both men and women. If this happens, discuss this with the radiation oncologist.

- **Questions about when to have intercourse.** Sometimes people are reluctant to talk about their sexual activities. However, it is best to be open and to ask the doctor or nurse about when to resume intercourse. It is also important to ask about symptoms that may be a sign to stop intercourse.
- **A sexual partner is fearful.** Some partners may want to resume sexual activity but are afraid because they fear they will hurt the person with cancer, spread the cancer, or even get cancer themselves. Talking about these concerns with doctors and nurses can be helpful. Cancer is not contagious and it will not spread through sexual activity.
- **Concern because of having little or no interest in sexual activities or feelings.** If the person with cancer or the partner is concerned about having little interest in sexual intercourse, discussing the problem with a doctor or nurse can help. They will explain the causes and when sexual interest may be expected to return.
- **Inability or unwillingness to talk about changes in sexual activities or feelings, even when asked.** Talking about sexual issues can be difficult, especially if the person with cancer has not talked openly about sex in the past, feels unattractive, or does not want to admit to having sexual problems.
- **Questions about wanting to become pregnant.** Usually pregnancy is avoided during chemotherapy treatments and adequate birth control is necessary.

Note that not all professionals will be knowledgeable about these issues. Therefore, if the first professional you talk to can't help, keep looking. Ask for a referral to a professional counselor who has experience helping people with these problems.

What You Can Do to Help

Women with cancer

Treatments and surgery in the pelvic or abdominal area can change sexual responses or a woman's willingness to touch intimately. For example, women who have had hysterectomies, urinary surgery, or surgery that increases the likelihood of urine leaking can benefit from these suggestions.

Empty the bladder before intercourse or before touching. Muscles around the opening to the vagina may have been weakened by surgery. The opening to the tube that carries urine out of the body may also have been weakened. Emptying the bladder before sexual touching or intercourse decreases the chance of urine leaking out.

Empty the bladder before any type of sexual activity if the woman is catheterizing herself to drain urine. Some women, whose urinary system has been injured after surgery or because of cancer, may need to self-catheterize every few hours to remove urine from the bladder. They may have to do this for a short time or permanently. In either case, it is wise to self-catheterize before any sexual activity. Feelings of fullness in the bladder can interfere with feelings of sexual relaxation and pleasure.

Lubricate the vagina with a water-based gel before sexual activity. Some cancer treatments make the vagina drier, which may cause a delay in making fluids that aid intercourse. Vaginal dryness can also happen because of aging or general worry about having sex. Dryness can be caused by medicines, including some chemotherapies, by radiation treatment, and by surgery. Dryness can be treated by lubricating the vagina with a water-based gel before sexual activity. Some brands can be used a few times during the week to help soften and moisturize the vagina and outside skin; these brands do not have to be used every day or every time before intercourse. For best results, avoid petroleum jelly and look for a gel that does not have an alcohol base.

Learn what changes to expect in sexual feelings and responses and how long these changes will last if the person with cancer is taking hormones for cancer. Sometimes, antiestrogens are prescribed to reduce the risk of getting breast cancer again, but they may have side effects such as shakiness or hot flashes. Find out when side effects may appear, how long they will last, and when they will disappear. Also, ask how antiestrogens may affect vaginal wetness or feelings of desire and excitement. The doctor or nurse can tell you what these drugs do and what side effects to expect.

Learn what changes to expect in sexual feelings and responses and how long these changes will last if the person with cancer is receiving chemotherapy or radiotherapy. Some chemotherapy medicines and radiotherapy treatments cause changes in vaginal wetness and in normal sexual responses. Ask the nurse or doctor about this.

Call the American Cancer Society and ask a Reach to Recovery® volunteer to visit if the person with cancer has had a mastectomy, lumpectomy, or postmastectomy reconstruction for breast cancer. Your local American Cancer Society will assign a volunteer who has had breast cancer, surgery, and treatment. These volunteers visit the person with cancer in the hospital and at home. They demonstrate arm exercises to do after surgery, explain what to expect in healing and using the arm on the surgical side, and discuss dressing, bras, and breast prostheses. They can also answer questions about sexuality, feeling attractive, and sexual activities.

Find out if the cancer treatments cause infertility (not being able to have a child). Some cancer surgeries or treatments result in female infertility. For example, when the ovaries or uterus are removed, a woman can no longer have a child. High-dose radiation may also result in infertility.

Men with cancer

Ask if "dry orgasms" will happen. When a man has the feeling of an orgasm but does not ejaculate, it is called a "dry orgasm." Certain surgeries and treatments cause more sex-related nerve and blood vessel damage than others. Nerve and blood vessel injury near the penis or prostate, or in the pelvic area, changes the way men experience desire, erections, and orgasms. They can also affect whether they continue to ejaculate.

Find out if banking sperm is an option if the man with cancer might want to father children in the future. Some cancer surgeries and treatments, such as removal of the testicles or high-dose radiation therapy, especially in the genital area, result in sterility. If you or the person with cancer are concerned about sterility, ask the doctor about banking sperm, especially if there is even the slight possibility that he may want to be a future father. Sperm is collected by the man before the surgery or treatment and frozen (or "banked") for future use, when it can be implanted through artificial insemination in a woman's womb to make her pregnant.

Learn what changes to expect and how long they will last if the person with cancer is taking hormone drugs as a cancer treatment. Sometimes, the level of testosterone falls after cancer surgery or treatments. A low testosterone level can cause problems with erections and even lower sexual desire. The doctor can check testosterone blood levels, and, if they are too low, additional testosterone drug doses can be ordered. However, in the case of prostate cancer, male hormones are not given because they can speed up the growth of prostate cancer.

Ask about the side effects of DES if the person with cancer is taking this hormone. Be sure that you and he know about its expected side effects and when they will appear, including how DES may change sexual responses such as erections or feelings of desire.

Ask about penis implants (also called penile implants) and other options if erections may be a problem after treatment or surgery. If the man with cancer wants to have more success with erections, penile implants or prostheses are an option. Some create a permanent or semirigid erection that can be hidden under clothes. Other implants are inflatable, which gives a man more control over when to have an erection. In this case, a small pump is placed under the skin, and the erection occurs because the man pushes the pump several times, usually to let water fill tubes placed inside the penis. Other types of implants and options are also available. Surgeons and urologists know about the options and can discuss the pros and cons of each with the person with cancer and his sexual partner.

Help the person with cancer prevent infection from sexual contact

Infections can happen from sexual contact when the immune system is functioning poorly as a result of chemotherapy or radiotherapy treatments. Here are some things that can be done to prevent infections:

Wash hands before and after sexual contact and after using the bathroom. Thorough hand washing is the most important way to prevent infection caused by touching the genitals and caressing.

Urinate after sex. Urinating after sex rinses out bacteria that may cause infection. After sexual activity, new bacteria are left near the urinary tract. Should the immune system be impaired, these bacteria can lead to an infection, not just in the urinary tract but elsewhere too. Ask the doctor whether the person with cancer risks infection more than usual by having sexual contact.

Avoid sexual contact with people who may have infectious and transmissible diseases like colds, flu, or cold sores. This includes all infectious diseases, from colds to sexually transmitted diseases, including AIDS. Condoms can help prevent the spread of infectious diseases, but they are not 100 percent effective for all infections. If condoms are used, use water-based lubricant on the outside of the condom. Do not use oil-based lubricants, such as petroleum jelly, shortening, mineral oil, massage oils, or body lotions, since they can cause the condom to break.

Clean the rectum thoroughly after bowel movements. Infections are easily spread from bacteria around the anus to the opening of the vagina or penis. The best way to prevent this is to gently wash the anus and surrounding skin with warm water and soap.

Possible Obstacles

Here are obstacles other people have faced in dealing with sexual problems from cancer:

"Who would think of sex at a time like this?"

Sexual feelings and thoughts can happen anytime, and it is normal to have them. They may be caused by a need for being close and for being held, and for feeling loved, secure, and accepted. Sexual activities may also distract a person from worries.

"He is concerned about sex, but doesn't want to talk about it."

You can mention to the doctor or nurse that he or she is concerned about sex, and they can raise the issue when talking with the person. You can also ask about whether a sex therapist works in your area. These professionals specialize in helping people learn or relearn how to enjoy sexual contact. Often their fees are covered by insurance if the visits are ordered by a doctor. Often only a few visits are needed to learn about what to do and how to cope with changes in sexual life.

"I am afraid to have intercourse or do anything like we used to do."

It may take time to try new ways of touching or having intercourse. Talk with a trusted health care professional. He or she will understand your concerns and help you with ideas on how to give and receive sexual enjoyment.

No matter how old a person is, being touched and held are important ways to show affection and feel comforted, even if you must postpone or give up intercourse.

Think of other obstacles that could interfere with carrying out your plan

What additional roadblocks could get in the way of doing the things recommended in this chapter? For example, will the person with cancer cooperate? Will other people help? How will you explain your needs to medical staff? Do you have the time and energy to carry out the plan?

Develop plans for getting around these roadblocks using the six problem-solving steps discussed in the first section of this book (see pages xi–xvi).

Carrying Out and Adjusting Your Plan

Carrying out your plan

Sex is a sensitive subject for most people. Think carefully about what you will do and especially how you will discuss the subject with the person with cancer. Be patient and let the person with cancer move at a pace that is comfortable for him or her.

Health professionals can be very helpful. They are often skilled in raising and discussing sexual matters. However, not all professionals are skilled or knowledgeable. Therefore, if the first professionals you talk to are not helpful with sexual problems, persist until you find ones that are.

If your plan doesn't work...

If sexual concerns remain a problem, your plan does not seem to be working, or these problems are happening more often, reread the section *When to Get Professional Help* (pages 255–256). If any of the conditions listed there exist, call the doctor or nurse for advice and a referral to someone you can talk with.

Tiredness and Fatigue

Understanding the Condition

Tiredness is a very common problem among people receiving treatments for cancer. People with cancer often say they feel more tired than ever before in their lives. There are some things you can do to reduce the tiredness—but you can also help the person with cancer make the best use of the energy he or she has. To do this, you need to work together as a team.

People receiving cancer treatments often may feel very worn out and tired. Tiredness may be caused by the disease itself or by the treatments. It may be caused by anemia, which means there are fewer red blood cells circulating oxygen to the body. Anemia can be caused by cancer, its treatments, or nutritional problems. Treatment depends on the cause of the anemia.

Other causes of tiredness are malnutrition (not eating enough) or a temporary increase in waste products as cancer cells are destroyed by cancer treatments.

Sometimes people feel tired after each course of treatment for their cancer. They complain of not having enough energy or not feeling like they can get going.

Tiredness may also happen because normal resting and sleep habits are disrupted. It may happen because the person with cancer is feeling depressed or in pain.

Try not to "push" the person with cancer to do more than what she or he feels is reasonable. Let him or her decide how much to do. If other symptoms occur with increased fatigue, then it's important to talk with the doctor or nurse.

Recent research suggests regular exercise may help to reduce fatigue. While more research is needed to be certain, some studies have shown that people with cancer who participate in regular exercise programs have better physical performance and less fatigue than those who do not. Exercise strengthens muscles and adds flexibility. It may also help combat depression. However, people with cancer should talk with their doctors or nurses before starting an exercise program. Exercise should not cause muscle strain or add to fatigue. Doctors and nurses who are familiar with the person's physical condition can judge if exercise would be helpful and, if so, how much.

Your goals for the person with cancer are to:

- call for professional help if it is needed
- help the person conserve energy
- promote sleep and rest

When to Get Professional Help

Tiredness, by itself, is not an emergency. However, some other symptoms that may occur in combination with tiredness are serious. When these symptoms occur along with tiredness, get immediate help.

Call the doctor or nurse if any of the following conditions exist along with tiredness:

- ▲ **Severe or frequent dizziness.** Dizziness, or feeling a loss of balance, can happen when walking, getting out of bed, or moving from a sitting to a standing position. Dizziness can also occur without moving or changing one's position. Dizziness can happen to anyone occasionally. When it is severe and frequent, get medical help. Severe dizziness can be caused by a drop in blood pressure, not eating or drinking enough, or other physical problems.
- ▲ **Falling followed by an injury, bleeding, mental confusion, or unconsciousness.** Report all bad falls so the doctor or nurse can judge what caused the fall, whether bones were broken, and what follow-up is needed. Sometimes they'll recommend using equipment to prevent future falls and may refer the person to a physical therapist or occupational therapist for evaluation.
- ▲ **Inability to wake up.** Call right away if you cannot wake up the person with cancer or if a sudden and unexpected change in the level of consciousness or alertness occurs. You will probably have to take the person to a medical facility for tests to determine the cause of this problem.

- **Feeling out of breath.** Breathlessness usually happens because the body is not getting the right amount of air and oxygen. This can be caused by a problem with the lungs and respiratory system or by a low level of red blood cells.
- **Feeling as if the heart is racing with minimal activity.**

When symptoms are not an emergency, but should be reported

Other problems that might appear with fatigue and should be reported during regular office or clinic hours include the following:

Ringing in the ears. This problem could be caused by a reaction to medicines, a change in blood flow to the brain, or other physical problems. Medical tests are usually required to determine its cause.

Pounding in the head. This could signal a problem with blood flow or blood pressure. Medical tests are usually required to determine its cause.

Staying in bed for days. Staying in bed can be a sign of depression if it continues for days on end without other symptoms. See the chapter *Depression* (pages 100–113) if this happens.

Know the following facts before you call the doctor or nurse:

- How clear are the person's thoughts compared with his or her thoughts before the symptoms happened? ________________

  ____
- Has any confusion appeared or increased since fatigue began?

  ____
- Is the person with cancer feeling depressed or "blue"? ________
- Has any new medicine been started, such as pain medicine or sleep medicine? ________________________________

Here is an example of what you might say when calling:

"My daughter is Dr. Harvey's patient. She feels some pounding in her head. She's been very tired lately, and today she complained of this pounding. She says it feels different from a headache."

What You Can Do to Help

If you decide that tiredness is not an emergency, there are things you can do to help manage this problem:

- help the person conserve energy
- promote rest and sleep

Help the person conserve energy

Plan the day's activities so being with people or trips happen when he or she feels most refreshed and awake. Allow time for rest between events.

Encourage resting between bathing, dressing, and walking.

Encourage doing things only for short periods of time. Break activities into parts that can be done for a short time. Also encourage resting ahead of time.

Agree on what's most important to do. Discuss which activities bring the most enjoyment or are necessary. Start with the most necessary or enjoyable activities, and don't be disappointed if all things on the list do not get done. Be realistic in the goals you set.

Encourage getting up or moving slowly to avoid dizziness. Dizziness can result from fatigue. When getting up from lying down, encourage sitting on the edge of the bed and dangling the feet and legs for at least four minutes before standing up.

Plan regular exercise to reduce fatigue. Plan to do something every day, even if it's as little as getting dressed or walking out to sit on the porch. Short walks are also helpful. Ask the doctor or nurse about a moderate exercise plan.

Serve a balanced diet with adequate protein. Serve from the four food groups (dairy products; fruits and vegetables; breads, cereals, rice, and pasta; and proteins such as meat, chicken, fish, or eggs). The most important food group is carbohydrates, which give the most energy. Examples of carbohydrates are pasta, potatoes, bread, fruit, and energy bars.

Ask relatives and neighbors to bring food, or call a community meals program to deliver balanced meals. Special menus are often available for people on low-sodium and diabetic diets.

Serve snacks as well as regular meals. Eating between meals is a good way to increase the amount of food eaten.

Promote rest and sleep

Encourage the person with tiredness to do some or all of the following:

Keep as active as possible during the day so that normal fatigue sets in at night. If the person with fatigue remains active throughout the day, then sleep is easier at night.

Include an exercise plan that is approved by the doctor. Regular exercise can have a positive impact on better sleeping habits as well as reducing stress, anxiety, and depression. Ask the doctor or nurse if they can recommend a program that will be suitable for the person's current condition.

Resume usual patterns of rest, and sleep as much as possible. Set regular times to nap and sleep, so the body comes to expect a routine. Routine habits help sleep.

Read the chapter on anxiety (pages 88–99) if nervousness or anxiety interrupts rest or sleep. It offers some good ideas on handling anxiety, including instructions on how to become relaxed. Talking with, touching, and listening to the person can also help.

Rest when tired by going to bed earlier, sleeping later, and taking naps during the day. If naps are a habit, then taking longer ones allows more rest and helps to reduce fatigue. Ask visitors to plan visits around sleeping and napping times.

Play relaxing music before sleep. Use whatever sounds helped to promote sleep before. Music or the sound of the television or of someone reading can be very soothing.

Use some type of relaxation exercise before bedtime. See pages 98–99 for a simple, effective relaxation exercise.

Drink warm milk at bedtime.

Take a warm bath or have a back rub at bedtime.

Ask the doctor about sleeping pills. If you have tried the other things on this list and the person with cancer is still having trouble sleeping, ask the doctor if sleeping medicine would help. Do not give sleeping medicine without checking with the doctor. These medicines can cause problems when combined with other drugs. Be sure the physician is aware of all other medicines being taken when you ask about sleeping pills.

Possible Obstacles

Here are some obstacles that have interfered with other people's plans for dealing with tiredness and fatigue:

"The fatigue comes with the treatments. There's nothing we can do to help it."

Cancer treatments often result in fatigue, but you can control how tiredness affects your life. There are also medicines to prevent anemia (low red blood cell counts), which the doctor can prescribe.

"There are so many things to worry about. No wonder I can't sleep."

Sleep often helps reduce anxiety because feeling tired can add to feeling anxious and jumpy. Set a goal of better rest as one of your top priorities. Set up a regular bedtime routine and do things to reduce stress at bedtime such as taking a warm bath, reading something pleasant, or spending time on a hobby.

Think of other obstacles that could interfere with carrying out your plan

What additional roadblocks could get in the way of doing the things recommended in this chapter? For example, will the person with cancer cooperate? Will other people help? How will you explain your needs to other people? Do you have the time and energy to carry out the plan?

Develop plans for getting around these roadblocks using the six problem-solving steps discussed in the first section of this book (see pages xi–xvi).

Carrying Out and Adjusting Your Plan

Checking on results

Keep track of how much of the day the person with cancer spends in bed. Check on whether current patterns of sleep and rest are similar to patterns before the illness.

If your plan doesn't work...

If your plan doesn't seem to be working, you may be expecting change too fast. It usually takes time to work out ways to live with tiredness. Try to set reasonable, realistic goals for what you can accomplish.

If tiredness is increasing and is of major concern to the person with cancer, ask the doctor or nurse for help. Tell them what you have done and what the results have been.

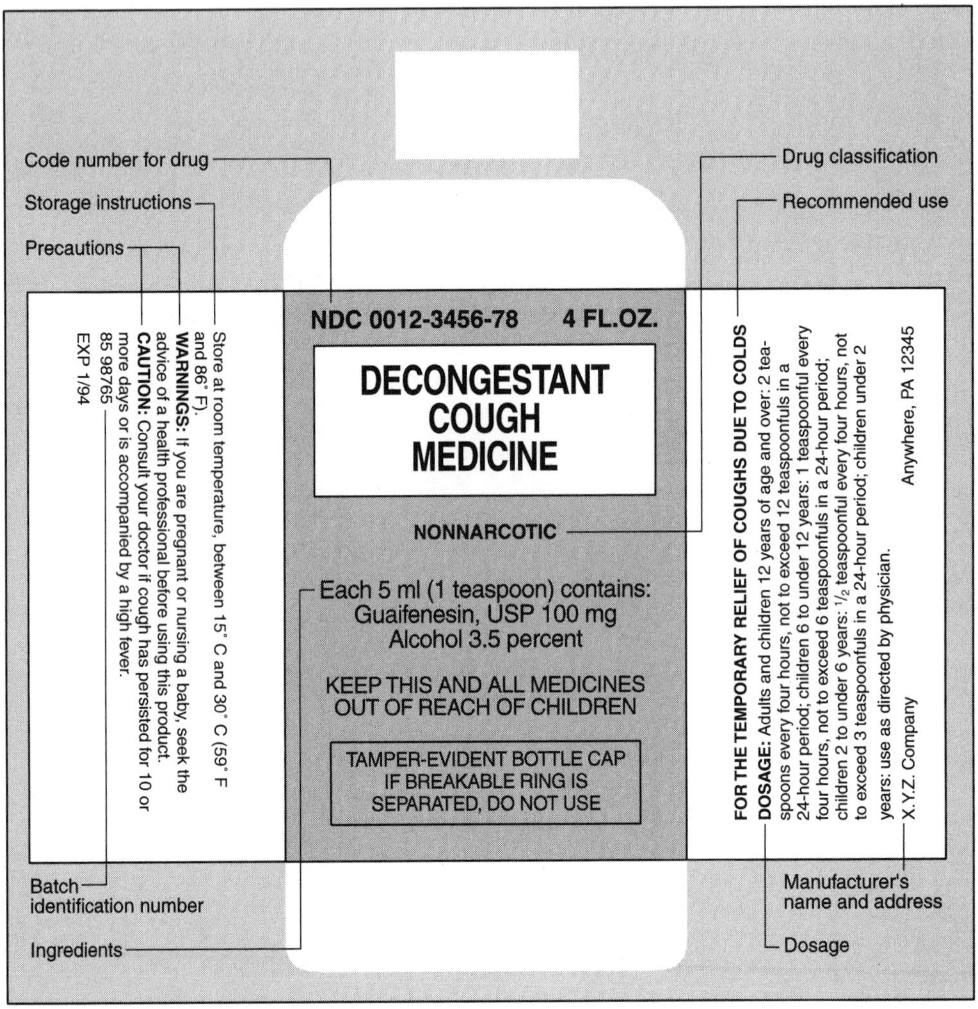

Code number for drug
Storage instructions
Precautions

Store at room temperature, between 15° C and 30° C (59° F and 86° F).
WARNINGS: If you are pregnant or nursing a baby, seek the advice of a health professional before using this product.
CAUTION: Consult your doctor if cough has persisted for 10 or more days or is accompanied by a high fever.
85 98765
EXP 1/94

Batch identification number
Ingredients

NDC 0012-3456-78 4 FL.OZ.

DECONGESTANT COUGH MEDICINE

NONNARCOTIC

Each 5 ml (1 teaspoon) contains:
Guaifenesin, USP 100 mg
Alcohol 3.5 percent

KEEP THIS AND ALL MEDICINES OUT OF REACH OF CHILDREN

TAMPER-EVIDENT BOTTLE CAP IF BREAKABLE RING IS SEPARATED, DO NOT USE

Drug classification
Recommended use

FOR THE TEMPORARY RELIEF OF COUGHS DUE TO COLDS
DOSAGE: Adults and children 12 years of age and over: 2 teaspoons every four hours, not to exceed 12 teaspoonfuls in a 24-hour period; children 6 to under 12 years: 1 teaspoonful every four hours, not to exceed 6 teaspoonfuls in a 24-hour period; children 2 to under 6 years: 1/2 teaspoonful every four hours, not to exceed 3 teaspoonfuls in a 24-hour period; children under 2 years: use as directed by physician.
X.Y.Z. Company
Anywhere, PA 12345

Manufacturer's name and address
Dosage

How to Read a Drug Label. Used with permission from *Nurse's Fact Finder*, 1991, ©Lippincott Williams & Wilkins.

Resource Guide

Cancer Information

AMC Cancer Research Center and Foundation

1600 Pierce Street
Denver, CO 80214
Toll-free Cancer Information and Counseling Line:
(800) 525-3777
Toll-free: (800) 321-1557
Phone: (303) 233-6501
http://www.amc.org

Through the counseling line of this nonprofit research center, you can request free publications and receive answers to questions about cancer. The Web site contains an area about ongoing research and general information about specific types of cancer.

American Cancer Society (ACS)

Toll-free: (800) ACS-2345
http://www.cancer.org

ACS is the nationwide, community-based, voluntary health organization dedicated to eliminating cancer as a major health problem by preventing cancer, saving lives, and diminishing suffering from cancer through research, education, advocacy, and service. The ACS offers up-to-date cancer information 24 hours a day, seven days a week. They also offer a wide variety of educational programs, services, and referrals. *Spanish materials are available.*

National Cancer Institute (NCI)

NCI Public Inquiries Office
Building 31, Room 10A03
31 Center Drive, MSC 2580
Bethesda, MD 20892-2580
Toll-free Cancer Information Service: (800) 4-CANCER
Toll-free (TYY): (800) 332-8615
http://www.cancer.gov

NCI is a federally funded government agency (part of the National Institutes of Health) that provides information on cancer research, diagnosis, and treatment to people with cancer, caregivers, and health care providers. It also maintains a listing of current clinical trials. The Cancer Information Service provides information to consumers and health care professionals. The Web site contains pamphlets and brochures on cancer diagnosis, treatment, research, and prevention. The NCI also maintains a listing of current clinical trials and other resources that may be helpful. It can also provide free pamphlets on various forms of cancer treatment, medication, clinical trials, and other cancer-related information. *Spanish-speaking staff and Spanish materials are available.*

National Comprehensive Cancer Network (NCCN)

50 Huntingdon Pike, Suite 200
Rockledge, PA 19046
Toll-free: (888) 909-NCCN (800-909-6226)
Phone: (215) 728-4788
Fax: (215) 728-3877
http://www.nccn.org

The NCCN is a nonprofit organization that is an alliance of cancer centers. The ACS has partnered with NCCN to translate the NCCN Clinical Practice Guidelines into a patient-friendly resource. The guidelines offer easy-to-understand information for patients and family members about treatment options for each stage of cancer. The treatment guidelines for patients are available for breast, prostate, lung, colon and rectal, ovarian, and melanoma cancer; the supportive care guidelines include nausea and vomiting, fever and neutropenia, cancer-related fatigue, and cancer pain. More guidelines are currently being developed. Call ACS for the latest guidelines, or view them online at either www.cancer.org or www.nccn.org. *Guidelines are also available in Spanish.*

OncoLink

Oncolink Editorial Board
University of Pennsylvania Cancer Center
3400 Spruce Street - 2 Donner
Philadelphia, PA 19104-4283
Fax: (215) 349-5445
http://www.oncolink.com

OncoLink is a service provided by the University of Pennsylvania and the University of Pennsylvania Cancer Center. Its mission is to help people with cancer, families, health care professionals, and the general public find accurate cancer-related information free of charge. The Web site provides information on cancer including clinical trials, support groups, educational materials, cancer screening and prevention, financial questions, and other resources for people with cancer.

Caregiver Resources

Family Caregiver Alliance

690 Market Street, Suite 600
San Francisco, CA 94104
Phone: (415) 434-3388
Fax: (415) 434-3508
http://www.caregiver.org

The Family Caregiver Alliance provides information and resources on long-term care. They also offer fact sheets, statistics, public policy statements, an online support group, and other links.

National Alliance for Caregiving (NAC)

4720 Montgomery Lane, Suite 642
Bethesda, MD 20814
http://www.caregiving.org

The NAC provides support to family caregivers and the professionals who help them and to increasing public awareness of issues facing family caregiving. They provide advocacy information to increase public awareness of issues facing family caregiving. Their Web site offers tips for caregivers, research reports, and caregiving product reviews.

National Family Caregivers Association (NFCA)

10400 Connecticut Avenue, Suite 500
Kensington, MD 20895-3944
Toll-free: (800) 896-3650
Fax: (301) 942-2302
http://www.nfcacares.org

The NFCA is a national, nonprofit membership association whose mission is to support family caregivers through education and advocacy. It offers information and education, support, public awareness, and advocacy. The NFCA provides referrals to national resources for caregivers and offers a bereavement kit for caregivers and related publications for a fee. The NFCA Web site also provides a report on the status of family caregivers and ten tips for family caregivers.

National Respite Locator Service

ARCH National Respite Network and Resource Center
Chapel Hill Training-Outreach Project
800 Eastowne Drive, Suite 105
Chapel Hill, NC 27514
Toll-free: (800) 7-RELIEF (or 800-773-5433)
http://www.chtop.com/locator.htm

Respite, a break for caregivers and families, is a service in which temporary care is provided to a child or adult with disabilities, or chronic or terminal illnesses, and to persons at risk of abuse and neglect. The National Respite Locator Service helps parents, caregivers, and professionals find respite services in their state and local area.

Well Spouse Foundation

63 West Main Street, Suite H
Freehold, NJ 07728
Toll-free: (800) 838-0879
Phone: (212) 685-8815
Fax: (212) 685-8676
http://www.wellspouse.org

The Well Spouse Foundation is a national organization that provides support to partners of the chronically ill and/or disabled. They offer letter writing support groups, a bimonthly newsletter, annual conferences, and weekend meetings. They also make referrals to local support groups throughout the country. The organization is involved with other groups in educating health care professionals, politicians and the public about the needs of "well spouses," and the importance of long-term care.

Wellness Community

919 Eighteenth Street, NW, Suite 54
Washington, DC 20006
Toll-free: (888) 793-WELL (888-793-9355)
Phone: (202) 659-9709
Fax: (202) 659-9301
http://www.wellness-community.org

The Wellness Community is a national nonprofit organization dedicated to providing support, education, and hope to people with cancer and their loved ones. Through participation in professionally led support groups, education workshops, nutrition and exercise programs, and mind/body classes, people affected by cancer can learn skills that enable them to regain control, reduce isolation, and restore hope regardless of the stage of their disease. The Wellness Community has 22 facilities nationwide, 14 satellites, 2 facilities abroad, and 6 additional facilities currently in development. All services are free of charge and are provided in a comfortable, home-like setting. The Web site has a wide range of patient education materials, information about local programs and services, online support groups, and more.

Home Health Care

American Association of Retired Persons (AARP)

601 E Street, NW
Washington, DC 20049
Toll-free: (800) 424-3410
Phone: (202) 434-3470
Fax: (202) 434-6483
http://www.aarp.org

The AARP is a membership organization that is committed to providing older adults with information on health care treatment, home care, caregiving, managed care, assisted living, insurance benefits, and resources. They also provide community service, publications, education, and advocacy. Membership is open to anyone 50 years old or older. *Spanish-speaking staff and Spanish materials are available.*

Centers for Medicare and Medicaid Services (CMS)

Department of Health and Human Services
7500 Security Boulevard
Baltimore, MD 21244-1850
Toll-free: (877) 267-2323
Phone: (410) 786-3000
TYY: (866) 226-1819;
TYY Phone: (410) 786-0727
http://cms.hhs.gov

The CMS is a federal agency within the U.S. Department of Health and Human Services that runs the Medicare and Medicaid programs—two national health care programs that benefit about 75 million Americans.

Medicare
8115 Kune Road
Indianapolis, IN 46250-04623
Medicare Hotline: (800) MEDICAR
(800-633-4227)
TTY/TDD: (877) 486-2048
http://www.medicare.gov

The toll-free help line answers questions and provides literature on Medicare, gives referrals to state Medicare offices, and gives referrals to local HMOs, which have contracts with Medicare. The Web site provides publications online, frequently asked questions, information on fraud or abuse, and other information. *Spanish-speaking staff is available.*

Emergency Investigational New Drug (IND) Program – Compassionate Use

Center for Drug Evaluation and Research (CDER)
Food and Drug Administration (FDA)—Cancer Liaison Program
HFD-150
5600 Fishers Lane
Rockville, MD 20857
Toll-free: (888) INFO-FDA (888-463-6332)
Phone: (301) 594-2473 (for the Review Division of CDER Oncology Drug Products)
Fax: (301) 594-0499
http://www.fda.gov/cder

People with cancer not eligible for clinical trials and in an immediate medical crisis may be able to receive drugs not yet approved by the FDA by having their doctor apply to the FDA for an Emergency IND. The contact information above is only for patients with cancer.

Health.gov

U.S. Department of Health and Human Services
Office of Disease Prevention and Health Promotion
http://www.health.gov

Health.gov is a portal to the Web sites of a number of multi-agency health initiatives and activities of the U.S. Department of Health and Human Services and other Federal departments and agencies. The Web site also has a link to healthfinder.gov, a guide to reliable consumer health information from the Federal Government, and the National Health Information Center (see below).

National Health Information Center (NHIC)
P.O. Box 1133
Washington, DC 20013-1133
Toll-free: (800) 336-4797
Phone: (301) 565-4167
Fax: (301) 984-4256
http://www.health.gov/nhic

NHIC is a health information referral service. It puts individuals with health questions in touch with organizations that are best able to provide answers. They maintain a database, accessible by Internet or telephone, with information on more than 1,100 health-related organizations and government offices that provide health information upon request. *Spanish materials are available.*

Health Insurance Association of America (HIAA)

1201 F Street, NW, Suite 500
Washington, DC 20004-1204
Toll-free: (800) 879-4422
Phone: (202) 824-1600
Fax: (202) 824-1722
http://www.hiaa.org

The HIAA is a trade association representing the private health care system in the United States. Its primary purpose is to advocate on behalf of the industry. The HIAA offers consumer information guides covering disability income, health insurance, long-term care, medical savings accounts, and publications covering all aspects of insurance. The toll-free number can be called for more information about state insurance agencies and for obtaining publications. The HIAA Web site provides consumer information online.

Job Accommodation Network (JAN)

President's Committee on Employment of People with Disabilities
P.O. Box 6080
Morgantown, WV 26506-6080
Toll-free: (800) 526-7234 for accommodation information or (800) ADA-WORK (800-232-9675) for information about the Americans with Disabilities Act
Phone: (304) 293-7186
Fax: (304) 293-5407
http://www.jan.wvu.edu

JAN offers information and counseling services to employers interested in learning how to hire, retain, or promote disabled persons, rehabilitation or placement professionals, and persons with disabilities. Trained counselors return calls within 24 hours. JAN provides information about the Americans with Disabilities Act. It will interpret the laws for the people with cancer, help them to determine the best ways to approach their employer, let them know their rights, and what accommodations to ask for. It can also refer the individual to the proper regulatory organization, if necessary. Listings of employment attorneys and adaptive equipment are also available.

National Association for Home Care (NAHC)

228 Seventh Street, SE
Washington, DC 20003
Phone: (202) 547-7424
Fax: (202) 547-3540
http://www.nahc.org

NAHC is the nation's largest trade association representing the interests and concerns of home care agencies, hospices, home care aide organizations, and medical equipment suppliers. It promotes and advocates for home care and hospice services, disseminates news and information, and provides a home care and hospice agency locator. The NAHC provides a state-by-state database of phone numbers for home care and hospice agencies. The Web site features an online Home Care/Hospice Locator and information for consumers about how to choose a home care provider.

National Consumers League (NCL)

1701 K Street, NW, Suite 1201
Washington, DC 20006
Phone: (202) 835-3323
Fraud Hotline: (800) 876-7060
Fax: (202) 835-0747
http://www.nclnet.org

The NCL protects the public by providing the consumer's perspective on concerns including medication information, privacy on the Internet, food safety, and child labor. The fraud hotline provides consumers with advice about telephone solicitations and how to report possible telemarketing fraud to law enforcement agencies.

Pharmaceutical Research and Manufacturers of America (PhRMA)

1100 Fifteenth Street, NW, Suite 900
Washington, DC 20005
Phone: (202) 835-3400
Fax: (202) 835-3414
http://www.phrma.org

PhRMA is a trade association representing research-based pharmaceutical and biotechnology companies that are devoted to researching and developing medicines that allow patients to live longer and more productive lives. This organization provides a *Directory of Prescription Drug Patient Assistance Programs* that contains information about how to make a request for assistance, what prescription medicines are covered, and basic eligibility criteria, all available online. Information about member pharmaceutical companies and drugs currently available, in clinical trials, or under development is also available. The Web site includes a database of new medications for cancer and other diseases, publications, and pharmaceutical issues.

Visiting Nurse Associations of America (VNAA)

11 Beacon Street, Suite 910
Boston, MA 02108
Phone: (888) 866-8773 or (800) 426-2547
Phone: (617) 523-4042
Fax: (617) 227-4843
http://www.vnaa.org

VNAA is a nonprofit association of independent Visiting Nurse Association (VNA) home health and hospice providers whose mission is to promote community based home health care. It provides services including skilled nursing and mental health care, hospice care, and home health care. The Web site contains a visiting nurse locator, caregiver and home care information, and related links to other organizations.

Hospice Care

Assisted Living Federation of America (ALFA)

11200 Waples Mill Road, Suite 150
Fairfax, VA 22030
Phone: (703) 691-8100
Fax: (703) 691-8106
http://www.alfa.org

ALFA is the largest association exclusively dedicated to the assisted living industry and the population it serves. They provide information about choosing an assisted living residence and publish a consumer brochure and checklist. They also offer a searchable online directory of assisted living providers.

Hospice Association of America (HAA)

228 Seventh Street, SE
Washington, DC 20003
Phone: (202) 546-4759
Fax: (202) 547-6638
http://www.hospice-america.org

Services: HAA is a nonprofit organization that provides leadership and advocacy in the development and application of hospice and its philosophy of care. This is a trade organization with one of the largest lobbying groups for hospices in the country. Through programs of professional development, research, public education and information, HAA assists those who cope either personally or professionally with terminal illness, death, and the process of grief. The HAA distributes general information about hospice to consumers on their Web site or in brochure format that can be ordered by telephone.

Hospice Education Institute/Hospicelink

3 Unity Square
P.O. Box 98
Machiasport, MA 04655-0098
Toll-free Hospicelink: (800) 331-1620
Phone: (207) 255-8800
Fax: (207) 255-8008
http://www.hospiceworld.org

This nonprofit organization provides general information and materials about hospice and palliative care and makes referrals to local programs. It does not offer medical advice or personal counseling.

Hospice Foundation of America (HFA)

2001 S Street, NW, Suite 300
Washington, DC 20009
Toll-free: (800) 854-3402
Phone: (202) 638-5419
Fax: (202) 638-5312
http://www.hospicefoundation.org

The HFA offers a broad range of programs for people with cancer, such as information and materials on hospice care, a hospice locator service, and educational programs. Their Web site has information on hospice and home care, HFA programs and materials, and links to related sites.

Hospice Net

401 Bowling Avenue, Suite 51
Nashville, TN 37205
http://www.hospicenet.org

Hospice Net is an independent nonprofit organization that works exclusively through the Internet. It contains more than 100 articles regarding end-of-life issues. Hospice nurses, social workers, bereavement counselors, and chaplains are available to answer questions via e-mail. The Web site has information about hospice care, bereavement, and a hospice locator service for both patients and caregivers.

Joint Commission on Accreditation of Healthcare Organizations (JCAHO)

One Renaissance Boulevard
Oakbrook Terrace, IL 60181
Toll-free: (800) 994-6610 (only to file a complaint about a health care organization)
Phone: (630) 792-5000
Fax: (630) 792-5005
http://www.jcaho.org

This nonprofit organization evaluates and accredits thousands of health care organizations in the United States, including hospitals, health care networks, and health care organizations that provide home care, long-term care, behavioral health care, laboratory and ambulatory care services. Performance reports of institutions and guidelines for choosing a health care facility are available to the public and can be obtained by calling the JCAHO.

National Association for Home Care (NAHC)

228 Seventh Street, SE
Washington, DC 20003
Phone: (202) 547-7424
Fax: (202) 547-3540
http://www.nahc.org

NAHC is the nation's largest trade association representing the interests and concerns of home care agencies, hospices, home care aide organizations, and medical equipment suppliers. It promotes and advocates for home care and hospice services, disseminates news and information, and provides a home care and hospice agency locator. The NAHC provides a state-by-state database of phone numbers for home care and hospice agencies. The Web site features an online Home Care/Hospice Locator and information for consumers about how to choose a home care provider.

National Hospice and Palliative Care Organization (NHPCO)

1700 Diagonal Road, Suite 625
Alexandria, VA 22314
Hospice Helpline: (800) 658-8898
Phone: (703) 837-1500
Fax: (703) 837-1233
http://www.nhpco.org

The NHPCO is a nonprofit membership organization that represents hospice and palliative care programs and professionals in the United States. The organization is committed to improving end-of-life care and expanding access to hospice care with the goal of enhancing the quality of life for people dying in America and their loved ones. The NHPCO provides information about hospice programs in local areas and other publications. The Web site contains related links, a hospice locator database by state, a newsletter, and other general information. It also has a discussion forum and other related links.

Patient and Family Support

American Association for Marriage and Family Therapy (AAMFT)

112 South Alfred Street
Alexandria, VA 22314-3061
Phone: (703) 838-9808
Fax: (703) 838-9805
http://www.aamft.org

This organization provides referrals to local marriage and family therapists. They also provide educational materials on helping couples live with illness and other issues related to families and health.

American Counseling Association (ACA)

5999 Stevenson Avenue
Alexandria, VA 22304-3300
Toll-free: (800) 347-6647
Toll-free fax: (800) 473-2329
Fax: (703) 823-0252
Phone (TDD): (703) 823-6862
http://www.counseling.org

The ACA provides information in the field of counseling and public fact sheets on coping with crisis.

Cancer Care, Inc.

275 Seventh Avenue
New York, NY 10001
Toll-free Cancer Care Counseling Line: (800) 813-HOPE
Phone: (212) 712-8080
Fax: (212) 712-8495
http://www.cancercare.org
Spanish: http://www.cancercare.org/espanol

A nonprofit social service agency, Cancer Care, Inc. provides counseling and guidance to help people with cancer, their families, and friends cope with the impact of cancer. The toll-free counseling phone number offers information, referrals, and support (for support, request to speak with a counselor or social worker). The Web site includes detailed information on specific cancers and cancer treatment, clinical trials, and links to other sites. The organization also provides videos, support groups (online, telephone, and face-to-face), workshops, seminars and clinics, a newsletter, and other publications to interested consumers. *Spanish-speaking staff is also available.*

Cancer Research Institute (CRI)

681 Fifth Avenue
New York, NY 10022
Toll-Free: (800) 99-CANCER (800-992-2623)
http://www.cancerresearch.org

An institute funding cancer research and providing public information on cancer immunology and cancer treatment, the CRI helps locate immunotherapy clinical trials and offers a cancer reference guide and other informational booklets.

The Candlelighters Childhood Cancer Foundation (CCCF)

P.O. Box 498
Kensington, MD 20895-0498
Toll-free information line: (800) 366-CCCF (800-366-2223)
Phone: (301) 962-3520
Fax: (301) 962-3521
http://www.candlelighters.org

CCCF is an international, nonprofit organization whose mission is to educate, support, serve, and advocate for families of children with cancer, survivors of childhood cancer, and the health care professionals who care for them. This organization helps families of children with cancer cope with the emotional stresses of their experience. CCCF holds regular meetings to discuss problems and exchange information. The organization works to gain local interest in the special concerns of children and their families. It serves as an information clearinghouse for children with cancer and their families.

City of Hope Pain/Palliative Care Resource Center (COHPPRC)

1500 East Duarte Road
Duarte, CA 91010
Phone: (626) 359-8111
Fax: (626) 301-8941
http://www.cityofhope.org/prc

The COHPPRC serves as a clearinghouse to disseminate information and resources to assist health professionals with improving the quality of pain management and palliative care. They offer information on a variety of topics including pain assessment tools, patient education materials, quality assurance materials, research instruments, and end-of-life resources. The Web site provides a list of publications and other materials available for order. Many publications are available online. *Spanish-speaking staff and Spanish materials are available.*

I Can Cope®

American Cancer Society (ACS)
Toll-free: (800) ACS-2345
http://www.cancer.org

This ACS program addresses the educational and psychological needs of people with cancer and their families. A series of eight classes discusses the disease, coping with daily health problems, controlling cancer-related pain, nutrition for the person with cancer, expressing feelings, living with limitations, and local resources. Through lectures, group discussions, and study assignments, the course helps people with cancer regain a sense of control over their lives. For more information or to locate an *I Can Cope* program in your area, visit "In My Community" on our Web site or call us toll-free at (800) ACS-2345.

Leukemia & Lymphoma Society (LLS)

1311 Mamaroneck Avenue
White Plains, NY 10605
Toll-free: (800) 955-4572 (for the Information Resource Center)
Phone: (914) 949-5213
Fax: (914) 949-6691
http://www.leukemia-lymphoma.org

The LLS is a national voluntary health agency dedicated to curing leukemia, lymphoma, Hodgkin's disease, and myeloma, and improving the quality of life of patients and their families. This organization was formerly known as the Leukemia Society of America (LSA). Patient service programs and resources available through local chapters of the LLS include financial assistance, support groups, one-to-one volunteer visitors (in some chapters), patient education and information, and referral to local resources in the community.

Look Good...Feel Better (LGFB)

American Cancer Society (ACS)
Cosmetic, Toiletry and Fragrance Association Foundation (CTFA)
National Cosmetology Association (NCA)
Toll-free: (800) 395-LOOK
http://www.lookgoodfeelbetter.org
Spanish:
http://www.lookgoodfeelbetter.org/index_7.00.html

In partnership with the CTFA, the NCA, and the ACS, this free public service program is designed to teach women with cancer beauty techniques to help restore their appearance and self-image during chemotherapy and radiation treatment. *Information is also available in Spanish.*

Man to Man®

American Cancer Society (ACS)
Toll-free: (800) ACS-2345
http://www.cancer.org

Man to Man is a prostate cancer education and support program that offers community-based group education, discussion, and support to men with prostate cancer.

National Association of Area Agencies on Aging (N4A)

927 Fifteenth Street, NW, Sixth Floor
Washington, DC 20005
Toll-free: (800) 677-1116 for Eldercare Locator
Phone: (202) 296-8130
Fax: (202) 296-8134
http://www.n4a.org

The N4A is the umbrella organization for the 655 area agencies on aging (AAAs) and more than 230 Title VI Native American aging programs in the United States. N4A advocates on behalf of the local aging agencies to ensure that needed resources and support services are available to older Americans. The AAAs and Title VI programs and agencies coordinate and support a wide range of home- and community-based services, including information and referral, home-delivered and congregate meals, transportation, employment services, senior centers, adult day care, and a long-term care ombudsman program. N4A operates a toll-free nationwide telephone service called Eldercare Locator, which helps caregivers locate services for older adults in their own communities.

National Association of Social Workers (NASW)

750 First Street, NE, Suite 700
Washington, DC 20002-4241
Toll-free: (800) 638-8799
Phone: (202) 408-8600
http://www.naswdc.org

This organization is concerned with advocacy, work practice standards and ethics, and professional standards for agencies employing social workers. The Web site provides a national register of clinical social workers for local referrals.

National Coalition for Cancer Survivorship (NCCS)

1010 Wayne Avenue, Suite 770
Silver Spring, MD 20910
Toll-free: (877) NCCS-YES (877-622-7937) for material orders
Phone: (301) 650-9127
Fax: (301) 565-9670
http://www.canceradvocacy.org

The NCCS is a network of independent organizations working in the area of cancer survivorship and support. Its primary goal is to assure cancer care for all Americans and generate a nationwide awareness of cancer survivorship. NCCS serves as an information clearinghouse and as an advocacy group. It publishes *The Networker* quarterly. The Web site includes information about conferences, events, survivorship programs, and cancer resources.

Reach to Recovery®

American Cancer Society (ACS)
Toll-free: (800) ACS-2345
http://www.cancer.org

This program is designed to help patients with breast cancer cope with their diagnosis, treatment, and recovery. The volunteers from this program are women who have had breast cancer and are specially trained to share their knowledge and experiences in a supportive and nonintrusive manner. Ongoing support groups are available to help deal with the challenges of breast cancer. *Reach to Recovery* also provides early support to women who may have breast cancer or have just been diagnosed with cancer.

Rehabilitation

Caitlin Raymond International Registry

University of Massachusetts Medical Center
55 Lake Avenue North
Worcester, MA 01655
Toll-Free: (800) 726-2824
Phone: (508) 334-8969
Fax: (508) 334-8972
http://www.crir.org

The Caitlin Raymond International Registry is a resource for patients and doctors conducting a search for unrelated bone marrow or cord blood donors. The organization will perform a free international search for an unrelated bone marrow or cord blood donor. Patient and donor searches of the American Bone Marrow Donor Registry (not listed here) donor files are coordinated through the Caitlin Raymond International Registry.

International Association of Laryngectomees (IAL)

8900 Thornton Road, Box 99311
Stockton, CA 95209
Toll Free: (866) IAL-FORU (866-425-3678)
Fax: (209) 472-0516
http://www.larynxlink.com

IAL is a nonprofit voluntary organization composed of approximately 250 laryngectomee member clubs. The purpose of the IAL is to assist local clubs in their efforts toward total rehabilitation of laryngectomees. IAL programs include skills education for laryngectomees; a registry of alaryngeal (post-laryngectomy) speech instructors; the Voice Rehabilitation Institute, which trains laryngectomees and therapists; and educational materials.

National Association of Hospital Hospitality Houses, Inc. (NAHHH, Inc.)

P.O. Box 18087
Asheville, NC 28814-0087
Toll-free: (800) 542-9730
Phone: (828) 253-1188
Fax: (828) 253-8082
http://www.nahhh.com

NAHHH is a nonprofit association of more than 150 nonprofit organizations located throughout the United States that provide family-centered lodging and support services to families and their loved ones who are receiving medical treatment far from their homes. It provides information about hospital hospitality house facilities, including Ronald McDonald Houses and Hope Lodges. Services vary from facility to facility and are offered at little or no cost to the guests.

National Bone Marrow Transplant Link (NBMT Link)

20411 West 12 Mile Road, Suite 108
Southfield, MI 48076
Toll-free: (800) LINK-BMT (800-546-5268)
Phone: (248) 358-1886
Fax: (248) 358-1889
http://www.nbmtlink.org

The NBMT Link is a nonprofit organization that serves as an information center for prospective Bone Marrow Transplant (BMT) patients and as a resource for health professionals. NBMT Link provides peer support to BMT patients and their families over the telephone. The peer-support volunteers are BMT transplant survivors who have been specially trained. The Web site has information for donors and transplant patients.

National Lymphedema Network (NLN)

Latham Square
1611 Telegraph Avenue, Suite 1111
Oakland, CA 94612-2138
Toll-free: (800) 541-3259 (for recorded information)
Phone: (510) 208-3200
Fax: (510) 208-3110
http://www.lymphnet.org

The NLN is a nonprofit organization providing assistance to lymphedema patients, health care professionals, and the public by dissemination information on the prevention and management of lymphedema. *Some information is available in Spanish.*

National Marrow Donor Program (NMDP)

3001 Broadway Street, NE, Suite 500
Minneapolis, MN 55413-1753
Toll-free: (800) MARROW2 (800-627-7692) for general information
Fax: (612) 627-8195
http://www.marrow.org

NMDP is a nonprofit organization that maintains a registry of volunteer marrow donors and blood stem cell donors, drawing on a network of donor centers, collection centers, transplant centers, cord blood banks, apheresis centers, recruitment groups, and a Coordinating Center in Minneapolis, Minnesota. The Web site contains a BMT resource guide and a survivor's guide, both of which can be printed directly from your computer. Resources for health care professionals are also available.

tlc

American Cancer Society (ACS)
Toll-free: (800) 850-9445
http://www.tlccatalog.org

"*tlc*," or Tender Loving Care, is a "magalog" (magazine/catalog) that combines helpful articles and information with products for women coping with breast cancer or any cancer treatment that causes hair loss. Products include wigs, hairpieces, breast forms, prostheses, bras, hats, turbans, swimwear, and helpful accessories at the lowest possible prices. Profits are reinvested in the program or other ACS Patient Support programs. From the privacy of your own home and at your leisure, you'll be able to select products for your special needs that are sometimes difficult to find in your community.

United Ostomy Association (UOA)

19772 MacArthur Boulevard, Suite 200
Irvine, CA 92612-2405
Toll-free: (800) 826-0826
Phone: (949) 660-8624
Fax: (949) 660-9262
http://www.uoa.org

The UOA is a volunteer-based health organization dedicated to assisting people who have had or will have intestinal or urinary diversions. This organization has more than 400 chapters. They provide emotional support and rehabilitation programs, preoperative and postoperative visitation programs, networks for parents of children with ostomies, and produce several publications, such as the *Ostomy Quarterly* magazine.

Glossary

adjuvant: medicine used to enhance the effects of other medicines, treat symptoms that may increase pain, and provide pain relief.

adjuvant therapy: treatment used in addition to the main treatment. It usually refers to hormonal therapy, chemotherapy, radiation therapy, or immunotherapy added after surgery to increase the chances of curing the disease or keeping it in check.

allogeneic bone marrow transplant: see *bone marrow transplant.*

alopecia: hair loss. This often occurs as a result of chemotherapy or from radiation therapy to the head. In most cases, the hair grows back after treatment ends.

analgesic: medicine for mild pain relief, such as acetaminophen. See also *nonopioids, nonsteroidal anti-inflammatory drug (NSAID),* and *adjuvant.*

analog: a synthetic version of a naturally occurring substance. See also *LHRH analogs.*

androgen: any male sex hormone. The major androgen is testosterone. See also *testosterone.*

anemia: a condition in which a low red blood cell count causes a person to feel fatigued and have shortness of breath.

anesthesia: the loss of feeling or sensation as a result of drugs or gases. General anesthesia causes loss of consciousness ("puts you to sleep"). Local or regional anesthesia numbs only a certain area.

antiandrogens: drugs that block the body's ability to use androgens. See also *hormone therapy.*

antibiotics: drugs used to kill organisms that cause disease. Antibiotics may be made by living organisms or they may be created in the lab. Since some cancer treatments can reduce the body's ability to fight off infection, antibiotics may be used to treat or prevent these infections.

antibody: a protein produced by immune system cells and released into the blood. Antibodies defend against foreign agents, such as bacteria. These agents contain certain substances called antigens, and each antibody works against a specific antigen. See also *antigen.*

antiemetic: a drug that prevents or relieves nausea and vomiting, common side effects of chemotherapy.

antiestrogen: a substance or hormone therapy (for example, the drug tamoxifen) that blocks the effects of estrogen on tumors. Antiestrogens are used to treat breast cancers that depend on estrogen for growth. See also *hormone therapy.*

antigen: a substance that causes the body's immune system to react. This reaction often involves the production of antibodies. For example, cancer cells have certain antigens that can be found by laboratory tests; they are important in cancer diagnosis and in watching response to treatment. See also *antibody.*

anxiety: a mental state of uncertainty, fear, and nervousness resulting from a real or perceived threatening event or situation. Prolonged or severe anxiety can result in impaired day-to-day functioning. People with cancer and caregivers commonly experience anxiety and fear.

apheresis: also called leukapheresis, a less complicated process for harvesting peripheral stem cells for transplantation.

aromatase inhibitor: a drug that stops estrogen production.

autologous bone marrow transplant: see *bone marrow transplant.*

benign: not cancerous; not malignant.

biologic response modifiers (BRMs): naturally occurring substances in the body that change the interaction between the body's immune defenses and cancer, improving the body's ability to fight the disease.

biological therapy: also called biological response modifier therapy, immunotherapy, or biotherapy, a type of cancer treatment that boosts the body's immune system to fight against cancer or lessens the side effects of some cancer treatments; interferon is one example.

biopsy: the removal of a sample of tissue to see whether cancer cells are present. See also *core needle biopsy, excisional biopsy, fine needle aspiration (FNA), incisional biopsy,* and *needle biopsy.*

blood count: a count of the number of red blood cells and white blood cells in a given sample of blood.

bone marrow: the soft tissue in the hollow of flat bones of the body that produces new blood cells.

bone marrow transplant (BMT): a complex treatment that may be used when cancer is advanced or has recurred, or as the main treatment in some types of leukemia or lymphoma. An autologous bone marrow transplant uses bone marrow from the person with cancer. An allogeneic bone marrow transplant uses marrow from a donor whose tissue type closely matches that of the person getting the treatment. A syngeneic BMT occurs when the donor is an identical twin.

brachytherapy: also called interstitial radiation therapy or seed implantation, internal radiation treatment given by placing radioactive material directly into the tumor or close to it. See also *internal radiation* and *interstitial radiation therapy.*

breakthrough pain: pain that occurs between scheduled times for giving pain medicine.

cachexia: a profound state of general poor health and malnutrition (poor dietary intake).

cancer: a group of diseases that causes cells in the body to change and grow out of control. Most types of cancer cells form a lump or mass called a tumor. Cells from the tumor can break away and travel to other parts of the body, where they can continue to grow. This spreading process is called metastasis. See also *neoplasm.*

catheter: a thin, flexible tube through which fluids enter or leave the body, usually intravenous; for example, a tube to drain urine. A central venous catheter is one that is placed into a large vein in the body and remains there as long as it is needed. See also *peripherally inserted central catheter (PICC), intra-arterial catheter, intracavitary catheter,* and *intrathecal catheter.*

chemotherapy: treatment with drugs to destroy cancer cells. Chemotherapy is often used with surgery or radiation to treat cancer when the cancer has spread, when it has come back (recurred), or when there is a strong chance that it could recur. See also *systemic therapy.*

clinical trials: research studies to test new drugs or other treatments to compare current, standard treatments with others that may be better.

colostomy: an opening in the abdomen for getting rid of body waste (feces). A colostomy is sometimes needed after surgery for cancer of the rectum.

conditioning: treatment with high-dose chemotherapy with or without radiation therapy that is usually used before stem cell transplantation.

constipation: a condition that occurs when bowel movements happen less often than usual and when stools are hard or difficult to move. Constipation can be caused by medicines used to treat cancer, narcotics, emotional stress, changes in diet, and decreased activity.

core needle biopsy: the removal of a cylindrical sample of tissue from a tumor for microscopic analysis using a relatively thick needle.

corticosteroids: sometimes called steroids, any of a number of steroid substances obtained from the cortex of the adrenal glands. They are sometimes used as a hormone therapy or to reduce persistent nausea. See also *hormone therapy.*

cryosurgery: also called cryoablation, a surgical technique that uses liquid nitrogen spray or a very cold probe to freeze and kill abnormal cells.

curative surgery: removal of a tumor when it appears to be localized and there is hope of removing all of the cancerous tissue.

depression: also called clinical depression, a psychiatric disorder characterized by a lack of concentration, insomnia or oversleeping, loss of appetite, feelings of extreme sadness, guilt, helplessness and hopelessness, and thoughts of death. Some cancer medicines can cause symptoms of depression.

diagnostic surgery: surgery used to obtain a tissue sample for laboratory testing to confirm a diagnosis and identify the specific cancer.

diarrhea: liquid stools in which the bowel movements happen more frequently and feel more urgent.

diethylstilbestrol (DES): a synthetic form of estrogen. At one time, DES was the main form of hormone therapy for men with prostate cancer. See also *hormone therapy.*

dosimetrist: a health professional who plans and calculates the proper radiation dose for cancer treatment.

dry orgasm: in a man, the feeling of an orgasm without ejaculation.

edema: build-up of fluid in the tissues, causing swelling. Edema of the arm or leg can occur after surgery or radiation. See also *lymphedema.*

electrosurgery: a surgical procedure that involves the use of high-frequency electrical current to destroy cells.

emesis: vomiting.

endoscopy: inspection of body organs or cavities using a flexible, lighted tube called an endoscope.

enema: the injection of liquid, such as mineral oil, chemically treated water, or soap suds, into the rectum (lower bowel) for cleansing, for stimulating a bowel movement, or for other therapeutic or diagnostic purposes; a stool softener for relief of constipation.

engraftment: the beginning of the growth of transplanted stem cells in a recipient's bone marrow.

enterostomal therapist: a health professional, often a nurse, who teaches people how to care for ostomies (surgically created openings such as a colostomy) and other wounds.

estrogen: a female sex hormone produced primarily by the ovaries, and in smaller amounts by the adrenal cortex. See also *hormone replacement therapy* and *hormone therapy.*

excisional biopsy: a type of diagnostic surgery in which a surgeon cuts through the skin to remove an entire tumor for testing.

external radiation: also called external beam radiation, radiation focused from a source outside the body on the area affected by the cancer. It is much like getting a diagnostic x-ray, but for a longer time.

feces: solid waste matter; bowel movement, or stool.

fiber: dietary fiber includes a wide variety of plant carbohydrates that are not digested by humans. Fibers are classified as "soluble" (like oat bran) and "insoluble" (like wheat bran). Good sources of fiber are beans, vegetables, whole grains, and fruits.

fibrosis: formation of scar-like (fibrous) tissue. This can occur anywhere in the body.

fine needle aspiration (FNA): in this procedure, a thin needle is used to draw up (aspirate) samples for examination under a microscope. See *biopsy* and *needle biopsy.*

gastroenterologist: a doctor who specializes in diseases or conditions of the digestive (gastrointestinal) tract. For example, a person with severe diarrhea might consult this type of doctor.

gastrointestinal tract (GI tract): the digestive (or intestinal) tract. It consists of those organs and structures that process and prepare food to be used for energy; for example, the stomach, small intestine, and large intestine.

GI tube: a temporary or permanent tube inserted into a hole that goes directly into the gastrointestinal tract. If a person cannot swallow food, GI tubes are sometimes used to put a thick nutritious fluid into the stomach.

hematoma: a collection of blood outside a blood vessel caused by a leak or an injury.

home health nurse: a health professional who gives medications in the home, teaches patients how to care for themselves, and assesses their condition to see if further medical attention is needed.

hormone: a chemical substance released into the body by the endocrine glands such as the thyroid, adrenal, or ovaries. Hormones travel through the bloodstream and set in motion various body functions. Testosterone and estrogen are examples of male and female hormones. See also *androgen, corticosteroids, estrogen, luteinizing hormone-releasing hormone (LHRH), progestin,* and *testosterone.*

hormone replacement therapy: in women, the use of estrogen and progesterone from an outside source after the body has stopped making it because of natural or induced menopause.

hormone therapy: treatment with hormones, with drugs that interfere with hormone production or hormone action, or the surgical removal of hormone-producing glands. Hormone therapy may kill cancer cells or slow their growth. See also *antiandrogens, antiestrogen, aromatase inhibitor, corticosteroids, diethylstilbestrol (DES), estrogen, intermittent hormonal therapy, LHRH analogs, progestin,* and *total androgen blockade.*

hospice: a special kind of care for people in the final phase of illness, their families, and caregivers. The care may take place in the person's home or in a home-like facility.

hyperalimentation: giving nutrition other than as food, often intravenously. See also *GI tube.*

ileostomy: an operation in which the end of the small intestine, the ileum, is brought out through an opening in the abdomen. The contents of the intestine, unformed stool, are expelled through this opening into a bag called an appliance. See also *ostomy.*

immune system: the complex system by which the body resists infection by microbes such as bacteria or viruses and rejects transplanted tissues or organs. The immune system may also help the body fight some cancers. See also *lymphatic system.*

immunotherapy: treatments that promote or support the body's immune system response to a disease such as cancer.

impotence: not being able to have or keep an erection of the penis.

incision: a cut made in the skin with a knife.

incisional biopsy: a type of diagnostic surgery in which the surgeon cuts through the skin to remove a small part of a large tumor for testing.

incontinence: partial or complete loss of urinary control.

informed consent: a legal document that explains a course of treatment, the risks, benefits, and possible alternatives; the process by which people agree to treatment.

infusion: introduction of a solution into the body through a vein for therapeutic purposes, usually lasting 30 minutes or more.

intermittent hormonal therapy: a type of prostate cancer treatment in which hormonal drugs are stopped after a man's blood PSA level drops to a very low level and remains stable for a while. If the PSA level begins to rise, the drugs are started again. See also *hormone therapy.*

internal radiation: treatment involving implantation of a radioactive substance. See also *brachytherapy* and *interstitial radiation therapy.*

interstitial radiation therapy: a type of internal radiation (or brachytherapy) treatment in which a radioactive implant is placed directly into the tissue (not in a body cavity).

intra-arterial catheter: a catheter that delivers fluids directly into an artery to treat a specific part of the body.

intracavitary catheter: a catheter that is placed in the abdomen, pelvis, or chest.

intrathecal catheter: a catheter that delivers fluids into the spinal fluid.

intravenous (IV): a method of supplying fluids and medications using a needle inserted in a vein.

intravenous (IV) catheter: see *catheter.*

insomnia: the inability to sleep. In the person with cancer, insomnia can occur as a result of pain.

investigational: under study; often used to describe drugs used in clinical trials.

IV push: drugs delivered through a thin needle inserted into a vein, given over a few minutes. See also *infusion.*

laparoscopy: examination of the abdominal cavity with a long, slender tube (called a laparoscope) inserted into the abdomen through a very small incision, similar to endoscopy.

laparotomy: examination and biopsy of the abdominal cavity with a laparoscope, similar to laparoscopy, but the midline incision in the abdomen extends from the upper to lower abdomen. This may be done when there is uncertainty about a suspicious area that cannot be diagnosed by less intrusive tests.

laryngectomy: surgery to remove the voice box (larynx), usually because of cancer.

laser surgery: a type of surgery using laser (Light Amplification by Stimulated Emission of Radiation) light. Laser light is a highly focused, powerful beam of light energy used in medicine for precise and relatively noninvasive surgical work.

laxative: a food or drug that stimulates the bowels to move waste products out of the body. For the person with cancer, a laxative may ease constipation caused by pain medicines.

leukapheresis: see *apheresis*.

LHRH analogs: human-made hormones, chemically similar to luteinizing hormone-releasing hormone. They block the production of the male hormone testosterone and are sometimes used as a treatment for prostate cancer. See also *hormone therapy* and *luteinizing hormone-releasing hormone (LHRH)*.

luteinizing hormone-releasing hormone (LHRH): a hormone produced by the hypothalamus, a tiny gland in the brain, that affects levels of luteinizing hormone in the body and therefore affects testosterone levels.

lymphatic system: the tissues and organs (including lymph nodes, spleen, thymus, and bone marrow) that produce and store lymphocytes (cells that fight infection) and the channels that carry the lymph fluid. The entire lymphatic system is an important part of the body's immune system. Invasive cancers sometimes penetrate the lymphatic vessels and spread (metastasize) to lymph nodes. See also *immune system*.

lymph nodes: small bean-shaped collections of immune system tissue such as lymphocytes, found along lymphatic vessels. They remove cell waste and fluids from lymph. They help fight infections and also have a role in fighting cancer.

lymphedema: a complication in which excess fluid collects in the arms or legs. This often happens after the lymph nodes and vessels are removed from surgery, or injured from radiation or from a tumor that interferes with normal drainage of the fluid (such as after breast cancer treatments). This condition can be persistent but not painful. See also *edema*.

manic depression: also called bipolar illness or manic-depressive illness, a type of mental illness characterized by alternating episodes of mania (changing ideas, exaggerated sexuality, excessive happiness or irritability, and decreased sleep) and depression. See also *depression*.

medical oncologist: a doctor who is specially trained to diagnose cancer and treat cancer with chemotherapy and other drugs.

metastasis: the spread of cancer cells to distant areas of the body by way of the lymph system or bloodstream.

Mohs' surgery: also known as microscopically controlled surgery, a technique for removing cancerous tissue by shaving off one layer at a time until the analyzed tissue looks normal. This technique is used when the extent of cancer is not known or when the maximum amount of healthy skin needs to be preserved.

needle biopsy: removal of fluid, cells, or tissue with a needle for examination under a microscope. There are two types: fine needle aspiration (FNA) and core biopsy.

neoadjuvant therapy: a systemic therapy, such as chemotherapy or hormone therapy, given before surgery or radiation. This type of therapy can shrink some tumors, so that they are easier to remove.

neoplasm: an abnormal growth (tumor) that starts from a single altered cell; a neoplasm may be benign or malignant. Cancer is a malignant neoplasm. See also *tumor*.

nonopioids: mild to moderate pain relievers, such as acetaminophen, aspirin, and ibuprofen. Many nonopioids are over-the-counter (without a prescription) medicines. See also *analgesic* and *nonsteroidal anti-inflammatory drug (NSAID)*.

nonsteroidal anti-inflammatory drug (NSAID): a mild pain reliever, examples of which are aspirin and ibuprofen. Check with your doctor before using these medicines. NSAIDs can slow blood clotting, especially if you are on chemotherapy. See also *analgesic* and *nonopioids*.

nurse practitioner: a registered nurse with a master's or doctoral degree. Licensed nurse practitioners diagnose and manage illness and disease, usually working closely with a doctor. In many states, they may prescribe medications.

oncologist: a doctor with special training in the diagnosis and treatment of cancer. A surgical oncologist is a doctor who specializes in using surgery to treat cancer.

oncology: the branch of medicine concerned with the diagnosis and treatment of cancer.

oncology clinical nurse specialist: a registered nurse with a master's degree in oncology nursing who specializes in the care of people with cancer.

oncology social worker: a health professional with a master's degree in social work who is an expert in coordinating and providing nonmedical care to patients. The oncology social worker provides counseling and assistance to people with cancer and their families, especially in dealing with the nonmedical issues that can result from cancer, such as financial problems, housing (when treatments must be taken at a facility away from home), and child care.

opioids: narcotic drugs used to relieve pain, all of which require a prescription. Some examples include codeine, morphine, and fentanyl.

ostomy: a general term meaning an opening, especially one made by surgery. An ostomy is not a disease; rather, it is a change in anatomy that may be necessary as a result of a disease or condition. Not all ostomies are permanent. See also *colostomy, ileostomy, stoma, tracheostomy,* and *urostomy.*

palliative treatment: treatment that relieves symptoms, such as pain, but is not expected to cure the disease. The main purpose is to improve the person's quality of life. Palliative surgery is surgery performed as a treatment of complications of advanced disease and to correct a condition that is causing discomfort or disability.

peripheral blood stem cell transplantation (PBSCT): stem cells used for transplantation are usually obtained from the peripheral blood (bloodstream) by a procedure called apheresis (also called leukapheresis); this occurs before the patient is treated with large doses of chemotherapy or radiation. After treatment, the patient receives a transplant of stem cells to restore the blood-producing bone marrow stem cells. There are three main types of SCT—allogeneic, autologous, and syngeneic. See also *bone marrow transplant.*

peripherally inserted central catheter (PICC): a type of catheter that allows continuous access to large arm vein for several weeks.

plastic and reconstructive surgeon: a surgeon specializing in restoring appearance or in the reconstruction of removed or injured body parts.

platelet: a specific blood cell that plugs up holes in blood vessels after an injury. Chemotherapy can cause a drop in the platelet count, a condition called thrombocytopenia that carries a risk of excessive bleeding.

premalignant: also called precancerous, changes in cells that may, but do not always, become cancer.

preventive surgery: sometimes also called prophylactic surgery, surgery performed to remove a growth that is not yet malignant (cancerous) but is likely to become malignant is left untreated.

primary site or tumor: the place where cancer begins. Primary cancer is usually named after the organ in which it starts.

prn: as the situation demands; as needed—used in writing prescriptions or referring to taking medicines. (Latin for *pro re nata.*)

progesterone: a female sex hormone released by the ovaries during every menstrual cycle to prepare the uterus for pregnancy and the breasts for milk production (lactation).

progestin: a hormone produced in the ovaries; a hormone therapy that may be considered as treatment for advanced breast cancer after other hormone treatments have been tried. See also *hormone therapy.*

prognosis: a prediction of the course of disease; the outlook for the cure of the person.

prosthesis: an artificial form to replace a part of the body, such as a breast prosthesis.

protocol: a formalized outline or plan such as a description of what treatments a patient will receive and exactly when each should be given. See also *regimen.*

radiation oncologist: a doctor who specializes in using radiation to treat cancer.

radiation physicist: a health professional who makes sure the radiation therapy equipment is working properly and ensures the machines deliver the right dose of radiation.

radiation technician: a health professional who operates the radiation equipment and positions the person receiving treatment.

radiation therapy: also known as radiotherapy, x-ray therapy, and irradiation, treatment with radiation (high-energy particles or waves, such as x-rays, gamma rays, electrons, and protons) to destroy cancer cells. This type of treatment may be used to reduce the size of a cancer before surgery, to destroy any remaining cancer cells after surgery, or, in some cases, as the main treatment. See also *external radiation* and *internal radiation.*

radiation therapy nurse: a health professional who provides nursing care and helps the person with cancer learn about treatment and how to manage side effects.

rectum: the lower part of the large intestine leading to the anus.

recurrence: cancer that has come back after treatment.

regimen: a strict, regulated plan (such as diet, exercise, or other activity) designed to reach certain goals. In cancer treatment, a regimen is a plan to treat cancer. See also *protocol.*

rehabilitation: activities to help a person adjust, heal, and return to a full, productive life after injury or illness. This may involve physical restoration (such as the use of prostheses, exercises, and physical therapy), counseling, and emotional support.

remission: complete or partial disappearance of the signs and symptoms of cancer in response to treatment; the period during which a disease is under control. A remission may not be a cure.

restorative surgery: also called reconstructive, surgery used to restore a person's appearance or restore the function of an organ or body part.

risk factor: anything that increases a person's chance of getting a disease such as cancer.

secondary tumor: a tumor that forms as a result of spread (metastasis) of cancer from the place where it started.

sexual therapist: a mental health professional with special training in counseling people about sexual changes, problems, and communication (for example, after treatment for cancer).

side effects: unwanted effects of treatment, such as hair loss caused by chemotherapy and fatigue caused by radiation therapy.

simulation: the process a radiation therapist uses to identify the exact place on the body where the radiation will be aimed.

social worker: a person who helps people find community resources and provides counseling and guidance to assist with issues such as insurance coverage and nursing home placement.

staging: the process of finding out whether cancer has spread and if so, how far. There is more than one system for staging.

staging surgery: surgery performed to determine the extent of disease and how far it has spread.

stem cells: immature cells that eventually develop into blood cells that circulate in the body. Stem cells mostly live in the bone marrow, where they produce blood cells. They have the ability to change into different types of blood cells needed by the body.

steroids: see *corticosteroids*.

stoma: an opening, especially an opening made by surgery to allow elimination of body waste. See also *ostomy*.

stomatitis: inflammation or ulcers of the mouth area. This condition can be a side effect of some chemotherapies.

subcutaneous: located or placed just beneath the skin; for example, a central venous catheter.

supportive surgery: surgery used to help with other types of treatment, such as the delivery of pain medicine or chemotherapy (via a peripherally inserted central catheter).

surgery: the treatment of disease, injury, or disfigurement by way of an operation. Surgery is the oldest form of treatment for cancer and offers the greatest chance for cure. See also *diagnostic surgery, laser surgery, Mohs' surgery, palliative treatment, preventive surgery, restorative surgery, staging surgery,* and *supportive surgery*.

syngeneic bone marrow transplant: see *bone marrow transplant*.

systemic therapy: treatment that reaches and affects cells throughout the body; for example, chemotherapy. See also *neoadjuvant therapy*.

testosterone: a male sex hormone, made primarily in the testes. In men with prostate cancer, it can also encourage growth of the tumor.

thrombocytopenia: a decrease in the number of platelets in the blood; it can be a side effect of chemotherapy.

thrush: a treatable infection of the mouth or esophagus; a temporary side effect of chemotherapy or radiation therapy to the throat or chest area.

total androgen blockade: also called combination hormone therapy, combined androgen blockade (CAB), total hormonal ablation, total androgen blockade, or total androgen ablation, the combination of antiandrogens and orchiectomy (removal of the testicles) and LHRH analogs to block the body's ability to use androgens. See also *antiandrogens, hormone therapy,* and *LHRH analogs*.

tracheostomy: surgery to create an opening of the trachea (windpipe) through the neck.

transdermal skin patch: a method of drug delivery in which a skin patch is placed on the body (chest or back) and delivers medicine through the skin for up to 72 hours.

transmucosal administration: a method of drug delivery in which medicine is absorbed through the lining of the mouth (by putting it inside the cheek or between the cheek and gums). This method is usually used when a patient cannot ingest tablets or liquid because of difficulty swallowing.

tumor: an abnormal lump or mass of tissue. Tumors can be benign (not cancerous) or malignant (cancerous). See also *neoplasm*.

urostomy: surgery to divert urine through a new passage and then through an opening in the abdomen. In a continent urostomy, the urine is stored inside the body and drained a few times a day through a tube placed into an opening called a stoma.

venipuncture: the puncture of a vein, usually to draw blood or to inject a substance. See also *intravenous (IV)*.

x-rays: one form of radiation that can be used at low levels to produce an image of the body on film or at high levels to destroy cancer cells. See *radiation therapy*.

Index

Page numbers followed by "f" represent figures; those followed by "t" represent tables